Oct '15

Hypoglycemia in Diabetes

Pathophysiology, Prevalence, and Prevention

2nd Edition

Philip E. Cryer, MD

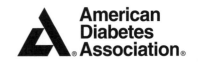

American Diabetes Association®

Director, Book Publishing, Abe Ogden; *Managing Editor*, Greg Guthrie; *Acquisitions Editor*, Victor Van Beuren; *Editor*, Rebekah Renshaw; *Production Manager*, Melissa Sprott; *Composition*, ADA; *Cover Design*, Koncept, Inc.; *Printer*, Thomson-Shore, Inc.

Printed in the United States of America
1 3 5 7 9 10 8 6 4 2

The suggestions and information contained in this publication are generally consistent with the *Clinical Practice Recommendations* and other policies of the American Diabetes Association, but they do not represent the policy or position of the Association or any of its boards or committees. Reasonable steps have been taken to ensure the accuracy of the information presented. However, the American Diabetes Association cannot ensure the safety or efficacy of any product or service described in this publication. Individuals are advised to consult a physician or other appropriate health care professional before undertaking any diet or exercise program or taking any medication referred to in this publication. Professionals must use and apply their own professional judgment, experience, and training and should not rely solely on the information contained in this publication before prescribing any diet, exercise, or medication. The American Diabetes Association—its officers, directors, employees, volunteers, and members—assumes no responsibility or liability for personal or other injury, loss, or damage that may result from the suggestions or information in this publication.

♾ The paper in this publication meets the requirements of the ANSI Standard Z39.48-1992 (permanence of paper).

ADA titles may be purchased for business or promotional use or for special sales. To purchase more than 50 copies of this book at a discount, or for custom editions of this book with your logo, contact the American Diabetes Association at the address below, at book-sales@diabetes.org, or by calling 703-299-2046.

American Diabetes Association
1701 North Beauregard Street
Alexandria, Virginia 22311

DOI: 10.2337/9781580404983

Library of Congress Cataloging-in-Publication Data

Cryer, Philip E., 1940-
Hypoglycemia in diabetes : pathophysiology, prevalence, and prevention / Philip E. Cryer. -- 2nd ed.
 p. ; cm.
Includes bibliographical references and index.
ISBN 978-1-58040-498-3 (alk. paper)
I. American Diabetes Association. II. Title.
[DNLM: 1. Hypoglycemia--physiopathology. 2. Diabetes Complications. 3. Hypoglycemia--epidemiology. 4. Hypoglycemia--prevention & control. WK 880]
616.4'66--dc23

2012031895

This book is dedicated to the research nurses, led for a

quarter of a century by Carolyn E. Havlin-Cryer, RN, and

the following research fellows:

Alan J. Garber, MD, PhD

William L. Clarke, MD

Alan B. Silverberg, MD

Steven A. Leveston, MD

Jack F. Tohmeh, MD

William E. Clutter, MD

Dennis A. Popp, MD

Ann M. Ginsberg, MD, PhD

Pierre Serusclat, MD

Thomas F. Tse, MD

Stephen G. Rosen, MD

Michael A. Berk, MD

Myrlene Staten, MD

David P. Hoelzer, MD

Natalie S. Schwartz, MD

Katherine R. Tuttle, MD

Karen M. Tordjman, MD

Stephen B. Liggett, MD

James C. Marker, PhD

Patrick J. Boyle, MD

Irl B. Hirsch, MD

Simon R. Heller, DM, FRCP

Brian V. Wiethop, MD

Samuel E. Dagogo-Jack, MB/BS

Dwight A. Towler, MD, PhD

Chatchalit Rattarasarn, MD

Annemarie Hvidberg, MD, PhD

Tarek Saleh, MD

Carmine G. Fanelli, MD

Deanna Paramore, MD

Fernando Ovalle, MD

Scott A. Segel, MD

Salomon Banarer, MD

Veronica P. McGregor, MD

Michael A. DeRosa, DO

Bharathi Raju, MD

Denise Teves, MD

Ana Maria Arbeláez, MD

Suzanne M. Breckenridge, MD

Benjamin A. Cooperberg, MD

Ranjani P. Ramanathan, MD

Nadia Khoury, MD

These individuals did the bulk of our work.

CONTENTS

PREFACE TO THE SECOND EDITION

Diabetes mellitus is an increasingly common disease. It is estimated that the prevalence of diabetes will rise from 285 million people in the year 2010 to 438 million people worldwide by the year 2030 (International Diabetes Foundation, 2009) and that the total diabetes prevalence (diagnosed and undiagnosed cases) will increase from 14% in 2010 to 25%–28% of the United States population by 2050 (Boyle et al. 2010). The common forms of the disease are type 1 diabetes mellitus, the result of absolute insulin deficiency from its clinical onset, and type 2 diabetes mellitus, the result of relative insulin deficiency in the setting of insulin resistance early in its course and absolute insulin deficiency later. Approximately 95% of affected people have type 2 diabetes.

Over time, diabetes can cause unique microvascular complications—retinopathy, nephropathy, and neuropathy—and a substantially increased risk for macrovascular atherosclerotic complications—myocardial infarction, cerebrovascular accidents, and peripheral vascular disease. These long-term complications are undoubtedly multifactorial in origin, but it is now well established, at least for microvascular disease, that hyperglycemia is one important factor. Maintenance of plasma glucose concentrations closer to the nondiabetic range prevents or delays microvascular complications in type 1 diabetes (Diabetes

Control and Complications Trial Research Group [DCCT] 1993; Diabetes Control and Complications Trial/Epidemiology of Diabetes Interventions and Complications Research Group [DCCT/EDIC] 2000) and in type 2 diabetes (U.K. Prospective Diabetes Study Group [UKPDS] 1998a, 1998b). It may reduce macrovascular complications in type 1 diabetes (DCCT/EDIC 2005; Polak et al. 2011) and type 2 diabetes (Holman et al. 2008). Indeed, it is conceivable that maintenance of normal plasma glucose concentrations over a lifetime of diabetes would eliminate the microvascular complications (DCCT 1995) and reduce the risk of macrovascular disease substantially (Stettler et al. 2006).

Unfortunately, with current treatment regimens, it is not possible to maintain euglycemia over a lifetime of diabetes in the vast majority of people with diabetes because of the barrier of iatrogenic (treatment-induced) hypoglycemia (Cryer 1997, 2004, 2008, 2010, 2011a). Pending the prevention and cure of diabetes, maintenance of euglycemia without hypoglycemia will require new treatment methods that provide plasma glucose–regulated insulin replacement or secretion, i.e. closed-loop insulin replacement, transplantation of β-cell containing tissue or expansion of β-cell mass.

The biochemistry, physiology, and pathophysiology of intermediary metabolism, with a focus on glucoregulation and hypoglycemia, have been reviewed (Cryer 1997, 2001, 2004, 2008, 2010, 2011a), and the history of hypoglycemia in the 20th century has been summarized (Cryer 1997). The impact of hypoglycemia was first documented in 1921 when a dog convulsed and then died after injection of extracted insulin; hypoglycemia was recognized to be a complication of insulin treatment of diabetes shortly thereafter (Bliss 1992).

Hypoglycemia is both a clinical and a physiological term. Unequivocal demonstration of clinical hypoglycemia requires documentation of Whipple's triad (Whipple 1938): symptoms, signs, or both consistent with hypoglycemia, a reliably measured low plasma glucose concentration, and resolution of those symptoms and signs after the plasma glucose level is raised (Cryer et al. 2009; Cryer 2011a). In healthy individuals, symptoms of hypoglycemia develop at an arterialized venous plasma glucose concentration of 50–55 mg/dl (2.8–3.0 mmol/l) (Cryer 2001). From a physiological perspective, however, the glycemic threshold is at a higher glucose level. Arterialized venous plasma glucose concentrations just below the postabsorptive physiological range, i.e., <70 mg/dl (<3.9 mmol/l), trigger physiological defenses against falling plasma glucose concentrations including further decrements in the secretion of insulin and initial increments in the secretion of glucose counterregulatory hormones such as glucagon and epinephrine (Cryer 2001). Indeed, the latter higher plasma glucose concentration, with or without symptoms, has been recommended as a pragmatic alert level for people with diabetes who are at high risk for clinical hypoglycemia (American Diabetes Association Workgroup on Hypoglycemia 2005; Cryer 2009).

This Second Edition of Hypoglycemia in Diabetes is updated and expanded but retains its focus on the clinical problem of hypoglycemia in diabetes. That problem is approached from the perspective of the pathophysiology of glucose counterregulation, the mechanisms that normally effectively prevent or correct hypoglycemia (Cryer 2001), in type 1 diabetes and advanced type 2 diabetes (Cryer 2004, 2008, 2010, 2011a).

The premise is that insight into that pathophysiology leads to understanding of the frequency of, risk factors for, and prevention of iatrogenic hypoglycemia in people with diabetes.

Philip E. Cryer, M.D.
Irene E. and Michael M. Karl Professor of Endocrinology
and Metabolism in Medicine
Washington University in St. Louis

ACKNOWLEDGMENTS

The author's original work cited has been supported in part by the U.S. Public Health Service, National Institutes of Health grants, including R37 DK27085, MO1 RR00036 (now UL1 RR24992), P60 DK20579, and T32 DK07120, and by research grants and a fellowship award from the American Diabetes Association. The author is grateful for the contributions of his mentors, collaborators, and colleagues; the efforts of the postdoctoral fellows who did the bulk of the work and made the work better by their conceptual input; and the skilled nursing, technical, dietary, and data management/statistical assistance of the staff of the Washington University General Clinical Research Center. Ms. Janet Dedeke, the author's valued assistant, prepared this manuscript.

DISCLOSURES

The author has served as a consultant to several pharmaceutical or medical device firms, including Amgen Inc., Bristol-Myers Squibb/AstraZeneca, Johnson & Johnson, MannKind Corp., Marcadia Biotech, Medtronic MiniMed Inc., Merck and Co., Novo Nordisk A/S, Takeda Pharmaceuticals North America, and TolerRx Inc. He does not hold stock in, receive research support from, or speak for any pharmaceutical or device firm.

Chapter 1.
The Clinical Problem of Hypoglycemia in Diabetes

THE CONTEXT

Iatrogenic hypoglycemia is the limiting factor in the glycemic management of diabetes (Cryer 2004, 2008, 2010, 2011a). First, it causes recurrent morbidity in most people with type 1 diabetes, and many with advanced (absolute endogenous insulin deficient) type 2 diabetes, and is sometimes fatal. Second, it compromises physiological and behavioral defenses against subsequent falling plasma glucose concentrations and thus causes a vicious cycle of recurrent hypoglycemia. Third, it generally precludes maintenance of euglycemia over a lifetime of diabetes and thus full realization of the microvascular and potential macrovascular benefits of long-term glycemic control (DCCT 1993; DCCT/EDIC 2000, 2005; UKPDS 1998a, 1998b; Holman et al. 2008). Hypoglycemia is not only common and potentially devastating; it is also costly (Quilliam et al. 2011).

Because of the barrier of hypoglycemia, no professional treatment guidelines recommend a glycemic goal of euglycemia, i.e., a normal hemoglobin A1c (A1C) level, although that would undoubtedly be beneficial with respect to the long-term complications of diabetes if it could be accomplished safely. For example, the American Diabetes Association (American Diabetes Association [ADA] 2012) recommends an A1C goal of <7% for many adult patients with diabetes.

Glucose is an obligate metabolic fuel for the brain under physiological conditions (Cryer 2001, 2007, 2010, 2011a). Mechanisms have evolved that normally very effectively prevent or rapidly correct hypoglycemia despite wide variations in glucose flux into and out of the circulation (Cryer 2001) (Chapter 2), undoubtedly because of their survival value. Thus, hypoglycemia is a distinctly uncommon clinical event, except in people who use drugs that lower the plasma glucose concentration, specifically insulin, a sulfonylurea, or a glinide, to treat diabetes (Cryer et al. 2009).

Clinical hypoglycemia is a plasma glucose concentration low enough to cause symptoms and/or signs, including impairment of brain function (Cryer et al. 2009). Because the clinical manifestations of hypoglycemia are nonspecific (Chapter 2), hypoglycemia is documented most convincingly by Whipple's triad (Whipple 1938): symptoms, signs, or both consistent with hypoglycemia, a low reliably measured plasma glucose concentration, and resolution of the symptoms and signs after the plasma glucose concentration is raised. However, because even asymptomatic low plasma glucose concentrations impair defenses against subsequent hypoglycemia (Chapter 3), hypoglycemia is defined more broadly in people with diabetes: all episodes of abnormally low plasma glucose concentration that expose the individual to potential harm (ADA Workgroup on Hypoglycemia 2005). Ideally, people with diabetes should self-monitor their plasma glucose level when they suspect it is low. However, because the risk of hypoglycemia is high in patients treated with insulin, a sulfonylurea, or a glinide—and the potential detrimental effects of untreated hypoglycemia outweigh those of unnecessary treatment—a clinical diagnosis of hypoglycemia is reasonable in such patients even in the absence of a glucose measurement, if the symptoms are compelling. Similarly, it is reasonable if a low glucose level is monitored, even in the absence of recognized symptoms.

Hypoglycemia in diabetes is generally the result of the interplay of relative or absolute therapeutic (exogenous or endogenous) insulin excess and compromised physiological and behavioral defenses against falling plasma glucose concentrations (Cryer 2004, 2008, 2010, 2011a) (Chapter 3). Thus, it is fundamentally iatrogenic, the result of treatments that raise circulating insulin levels and therefore lower plasma glucose concentrations. Those treatments include insulin or an insulin secretagogue such as a sulfonylurea (glyburide [glibenclamide], glipizide, glimepiride, or gliclazide, among others) or a glinide (nateglinide or repaglinide). Antidiabetic drugs, mostly insulin, were found to be second only to anticoagulants as a cause of emergency hospitalization for adverse drug events in people >65 years of age, and those visits were almost entirely because of hypoglycemia (Budnitz et al. 2011). Among other agents, sulfonylureas were found to consistently increase the risk for hypoglycemia more than metformin, thiazolidinediones, DPP-IV inhibitors, or a GLP-1 receptor agonist (Bennett et al. 2011). All people with type 1 diabetes must be treated with insulin. Most people with type 2 diabetes ultimately require treatment with insulin (Turner et al. 1999). Early in the course of type 2 diabetes, patients may respond to an insulin secretagogue, with the risk of hypoglycemia. Alternatively, they may respond to drugs that do not raise insulin levels at normal or low plasma glucose concentrations and therefore should not, and probably do not cause hypoglycemia (Bolen et al. 2007, Phung et al. 2010; Tschope et al. 2011). The latter include the biguanide metformin—which nonetheless has been reported to cause self-reported hypoglycemia (UKPDS 1995; Wright et al. 2006)—thiazolidinediones (e.g., pioglitazone, rosiglitazone), α-glucosidase inhibitors (e.g., acarbose, miglitol), glucagon-like peptide-1 (GLP-1) receptor agonists (e.g., exenatide, liraglutide, lixisenatide), and dipeptidyl peptidase-IV (DPP-IV) inhibitors (e.g., sitagliptin, saxagliptin, vildagliptin, linagliptin). All of these drugs require endogenous insulin secretion to lower plasma glucose concentrations, and insulin secretion declines appropriately as glucose levels fall into the normal range. That is true even for the GLP-1 receptor agonists and the DPPI-IV inhibitors, which enhance glucose-stimulated insulin secretion (among other actions). They do not stimulate insulin secretion at normal or low plasma glucose levels (i.e., they increase insulin secretion in a glucose-dependent fashion). However, the latter feature may be lost, and hypoglycemia can occur, when a GLP-1 receptor agonist or a DPP-IV inhibitor is used with a sulfonylurea (de Heer and Holst 2007). Indeed, all five categories of drugs—biguanides, thiazolidinediones, α-glucosidase inhibitors, GLP-1 receptor agonists, and DPP-IV inhibitors—increase the risk of hypoglycemia if used with an insulin secretagogue or with insulin. The bile acid sequestrant colesevelam and the dopamine receptor agonist bromocriptine should not cause hypoglycemia. Among potential future glucose-lowering drug categories, agents that inhibit renal glucose re-absorption (Ferrannini et al. 2010) or activate G-protein coupled receptor 40 (Burant et al. 2012) should not cause hypoglycemia, while glucokinase activators might well cause hypoglycemia (Bonadonna et al. 2010; Matschinsky et al. 2011).

FREQUENCY OF HYPOGLYCEMIA

If it is shown to accurately and reliably reflect plasma glucose concentrations and is linked to continuous recording of symptoms, continuous subcutaneous glucose monitoring might lead to more detailed knowledge of the precise prevalence and incidence of hypoglycemia in diabetes (Juvenile Diabetes Research Foundation [JDRF] Continuous Glucose Monitoring Study Group 2008; Cooke et al. 2009). Pending that, we must rely on estimates (Table 1.1).

Type 1 diabetes

Hypoglycemia is a fact of life for most people with type 1 diabetes (Cryer 2004, 2008, 2010, 2011a; DCCT 1993, 1997; U.K. Hypoglycaemia Study Group [UK Hypo Group] 2007; MacLeod et al. 1993; Donnelly et al. 2005; Reichard and Pihl 1994; Lüddeke et al. 2007) (Table 1.1). The average patient suffers untold numbers of asymptomatic episodes, two episodes of symptomatic hypoglycemia per week (thousands of such episodes over a lifetime of diabetes), and one episode of severe, temporarily disabling hypoglycemia, often with seizure or coma, per year.

Given increased recognition of the magnitude of the problem of iatrogenic hypoglycemia in type 1 diabetes, and practical improvements in the glycemic management of diabetes, over the nearly two decades since the Diabetes Control and Complications Trial (DCCT) was reported in 1993 (DCCT 1993), one might anticipate that hypoglycemia would have become less of a problem. Unfortunately, there is no evidence of that in population-based studies. For example, in their study reported in 2007, the U.K. Hypoglycaemia Study Group (UK Hypo

Table 1.1 Event Rates for Severe Hypoglycemia (That Requiring the Assistance of Another Person), Expressed as Episodes per 100 Patient-Years, in Insulin-Treated Diabetes

	n	Event rate	Comment
Type 1 Diabetes			
U.K. Hypoglycaemia Study Group 2007	57[a]	320	Prospective multicenter study
	50[b]	110	
MacLeod et al. 1993	544	170	Retrospective clinic survey, randomly selected sample
Donnelly et al. 2005	94	115	Prospective study, population-based random sample
Reichard and Pihl 1994	48	110	Clinical trial, intensive insulin group
DCCT Research Group 1993	711	62	Clinical trial, intensive insulin group
Type 2 Diabetes			
MacLeod et al. 1993	56	73	Retrospective clinic survey, randomly selected sample
U.K. Hypoglycaemia Study Group 2007	77[c]	70	Prospective multicenter study
	89[d]	10	
Akram et al. 2006	401	44	Retrospective clinic survey
Donnelly et al. 2005	173	35	Prospective study, population-based random sample
Henderson et al. 2003	215	28	Retrospective clinic survey, randomly selected sample
Murata et al. 2005	344	21	Prospective study, random Veterans Affairs sample
Saudek et al. 1996	62	18[e]	Clinical trial, multiple insulin injection group
Gürlek et al. 1999	114	15	Retrospective clinic survey
Abraira et al. 1995	75	3	Clinical trial, intensive insulin group
Yki-Järvinen et al. 1999	88	0	Clinical trial, initial insulin therapy
Ohkubo et al. 1995	52	0	Clinical trial, initial insulin therapy

[a]Insulin treatment for >15 years

[b]Insulin treatment for <5 years

[c]Insulin treatment for >5 years

[d]Insulin treatment for <2 years

[e]Definite (8 per 100 patient-years) plus suspected (10 per 100 patient-years) severe hypoglycemia

Studies covering at least 1 year, involving at least 48 patients, and reporting severe hypoglycemia event rates are included. This table was prepared, by the author, for a Clinical Practice Guideline on hypoglycemia in adults (Cryer et al. 2009).

Group 2007) found the incidence of severe hypoglycemia in patients with type 1 diabetes treated with insulin for <5 years to be comparable to that in the Stockholm Diabetes Intervention Study (Reichard and Pihl 1994) (both 110 per 100 patient-years) reported in 1994 and higher than that in the DCCT (Table 1.1). Remarkably, the U.K. Hypoglycaemia Study Group (UK Hypo Group 2007) found the incidence of severe hypoglycemia in patients with type 1 diabetes treated with insulin for >15 years (320 episodes per 100 patient-years) to be three-fold higher than in individuals treated for <5 years (Table 1.1). In addition, an incidence of 300 episodes per 100 patient-years was reported in 2007 in a prospective observational study of 7,067 patients with type 1 diabetes (Lüddeke et al. 2007). Indeed, a nearly 2-fold increase in the incidence of symptomatic hypoglycemia with a plasma glucose of <50 mg/dL (2.8 mmol/L) requiring treatment with intravenous glucose was noted from 1997–2000 to 2007–2010 in patients with type 1 and type 2 diabetes in one study (Holstein et al. 2012).

Hypoglycemia is particularly common during the night (Matyka et al. 1999; Raju et al. 2006). Nocturnal plasma glucose concentrations were <63 mg/dl (3.5 mmol/l) in 13 of 29 (45%) prepubertal patients with type 1 diabetes and the median duration of those low nocturnal glucose concentrations was 4.5 hours (Matyka et al. 1999). In adults treated with contemporary aggressive methods, and with relatively tight glycemic control, one quarter of all nocturnal plasma glucose concentrations were <70 mg/dl (3.9 mmol/l) and the duration of low values ranged up to seven hours (Raju et al. 2006). Six percent of the values were <50 mg/dl (2.8 mmol/l). The extent to which lower rates of nocturnal hypoglycemia detected in type 1 diabetes by continuous subcutaneous glucose monitoring (JDRF 2010) are a function of the monitoring technique or the patients studied is not known. However, that technique also did not distinguish patients with impaired awareness of hypoglycemia, who had a >3-fold increased incidence of severe hypoglycemia, from those with normal awareness of hypoglycemia (Choudhary et al. 2010).

Type 2 diabetes

Overall, hypoglycemia is less frequent in type 2 diabetes than in type 1 diabetes (UK Hypo Group 2007; Donnelly et al. 2005; Hepburn et al. 1993; Holstein et al. 2003; Leese et al. 2003) (Table 1.1). However, hypoglycemia becomes progressively more limiting to glycemic control later in the course of type 2 diabetes (UK Hypo Group 2007; UKPDS 1998c). Indeed, the frequency of hypoglycemia has been reported to be similar in patients with type 2 diabetes and patients with type 1 diabetes matched for duration of insulin therapy (Hepburn et al. 1993). When comparing patients with type 2 diabetes treated with insulin for <2 years with patients treated with insulin for >5 years, the U.K. Hypoglycaemia Study Group (UK Hypo Group 2007) found severe hypoglycemia prevalences of 7 and 25% and incidences of 10 and 70 episodes per 100 patient-years, respectively. The pattern for self-treated hypoglycemia was similar (UK Hypo Group 2007). Thus, while the risk of hypoglycemia is relatively low in the first few years of insulin treatment of type 2 diabetes (at least with current less than optimal glycemic goals), the risk increases substantially, approaching that in type 1 diabetes, later in the course of type 2 diabetes.

Because of the difficulty of ascertainment, reported incidences of hypoglycemia in diabetes are generally underestimates. Asymptomatic episodes of hypoglycemia will be missed unless they are detected by routine self–plasma glucose monitoring (or by reliable continuous subcutaneous glucose monitoring). Because the symptoms of hypoglycemia are nonspecific (Chapter 2), symptomatic episodes may not be recognized as the result of hypoglycemia (Clarke et al. 1995). Even if they are recognized, mild-to-moderate self-treated episodes are often not long remembered (Pramming et al. 1991; Pedersen-Bjergaard et al. 2003; Akram et al. 2009) and therefore may not be reported accurately at periodic clinic visits. Episodes of severe hypoglycemia (those sufficiently disabling that they require the assistance of another person) are more dramatic events that are much more likely to be recalled (Pramming et al. 1991; Pedersen-Bjergaard et al. 2003; Akram et al. 2009) and therefore reported (by the patient or by a close associate). Thus, although they represent only a small fraction of the total hypoglycemic experience, estimates of the incidence of severe hypoglycemia are the most reliable. (Arguably, they are also most important, since they pose a high risk for a subsequent serious adverse outcome and dictate consideration of a major change in the therapeutic regimen.) In addition, hypoglycemia event rates determined prospectively, particularly if hypoglycemia is the primary outcome in a population-based study, should be more reliable than those determined retrospectively.

While estimates of the incidence of hypoglycemia (Table 1.1) are often derived from clinical treatment trials, there are several limitations to that approach. First, hypoglycemia is not a primary outcome of such trials; therefore, the extent of collection of data concerning hypoglycemia varies. For example, much was learned about the incidence of hypoglycemia in type 1 diabetes in the DCCT (DCCT 1997), but the incidence of hypoglycemia in type 2 diabetes in the U.K. Prospective

Diabetes Study (UKPDS) is not known (Wright et al. 2006). Second, treatment trials in type 2 diabetes are often conducted in patients just failing oral hypoglycemic agent therapy and naive to insulin therapy. Such patients are not representative of advanced type 2 diabetes and are at relatively low risk for hypoglycemia, as mentioned earlier (UK Hypo Group 2007), for pathophysiological reasons developed in Chapter 3. Third, if used exclusively, that approach ignores evidence from clinical experience in diabetes specialist clinics and data from prospective, population-based studies focused on hypoglycemia.

The prospective, population-based study of Donnelly and colleagues (Donnelly et al. 2005) indicates that the overall incidence of hypoglycemia in insulin-treated type 2 diabetes is approximately one-third of that in type 1 diabetes (Table 1.1). In patients with type 1 diabetes, the event rates for any hypoglycemia and for severe hypoglycemia were ~4,300 per 100 patient years and 115 per 100 patient-years, respectively. In patients with insulin-treated type 2 diabetes, the event rates for any hypoglycemia and for severe hypoglycemia were ~1,600 per 100 patient years and 35 per 100 patient-years, respectively. Furthermore, in population-based studies from single hospital regions with known incidences of type 1 diabetes and type 2 diabetes, event rates for severe hypoglycemia requiring emergency medical treatment in insulin-treated type 2 diabetes were ~40% (Holstein et al. 2003) and ~100% (Leese et al. 2003) of those in type 1 diabetes. Because the prevalence of type 2 diabetes is ~20-fold greater than that of type 1 diabetes, and because most people with type 2 diabetes ultimately require treatment with insulin (Turner et al. 1999), these data suggest that most episodes of iatrogenic hypoglycemia, including severe iatrogenic hypoglycemia, occur in people with type 2 diabetes. Clearly, the magnitude of the problem of hypoglycemia in type 2 diabetes should not be underestimated.

In summary, compared with that in type 1 diabetes, the incidence of hypoglycemia is relatively low (at least with currently recommended glycemic goals) during treatment with an insulin secretagogue or even with insulin early in the course of type 2 diabetes (UK Hypo Group 2007). However, hypoglycemia becomes progressively more frequent, with its incidence approaching that in type 1 diabetes, in longstanding insulin-treated type 2 diabetes (UK Hypo Group 2007). As developed in Chapter 3, this increase in the frequency of iatrogenic hypoglycemia parallels progressive β-cell failure in type 2 diabetes and thus development of the pathophysiology of glucose counterregulation—compromised physiological and behavioral defenses against falling plasma glucose concentrations—as patients approach the insulin-deficient end of the spectrum of type 2 diabetes (Cryer 2004, 2008, 2010, 2011a).

IMPACT OF HYPOGLYCEMIA

Iatrogenic hypoglycemia causes recurrent morbidity in most people with type 1 diabetes and many with advanced type 2 diabetes and is sometimes fatal (Cryer 2004, 2008, 2010, 2011a). Because it generally precludes maintenance of euglycemia over a lifetime of diabetes, and thus full realization not only of the microvascular benefits (DCCT 1993, 2000; UKPDS 1998a, 1998b), but also of the potential long-term macrovascular benefits (DCCT/EDIC 2005; Holman et al. 2008), of glycemic control, the barrier of hypoglycemia may also contribute to the most prevalent cause of disabling morbidity and of mortality in diabetes—cardiovascular disease. Finally, hypoglycemia impairs defenses against subsequent hypoglycemia.

Morbidity

Glucose, almost exclusively derived from the circulation, is an obligate metabolic fuel for the brain under physiological conditions (Chapter 2). Hypoglycemia causes brain fuel deprivation that, if unchecked, results in functional brain failure that is typically corrected after the plasma glucose concentration is raised (Cryer 2007). Rarely, hypoglycemia results in death.

The physical morbidity of an episode of hypoglycemia ranges from unpleasant symptoms, such as palpitations, tremulousness, anxiety, sweating, hunger, and paresthesias (Towler et al. 1993), and cognitive impairments with behavioral changes, to seizure, coma, or, rarely, death (Cryer 2007). Physical injuries or transient focal neurological deficits occur rarely. Seemingly complete recovery after an episode of hypoglycemia is the rule. Permanent neurological damage is rare. In monkeys, 5–6 hours of blood glucose concentrations <20 mg/dl (1.1 mmol/l) were required for the regular production of overt brain damage (Kahn and Myers 1971).

It is conceivable that hypoglycemia, or more likely the responses to hypoglycemia, is a factor in the pathogenesis of macrovascular disease in diabetes. Patients with type 1 diabetes and recurrent severe hypoglycemia, compared with those without severe hypoglycemia, have been found to have lower flow-mediated brachial artery dilatation and increased carotid and femoral artery intima-media thickness, both markers of preclinical atherosclerosis (Giménez et al. 2011). Mechanisms by which responses to hypoglycemia might contribute to macro-vascular disease have been summarized (Younk and Davis 2011; Frier et al. 2011; Chow and Heller 2012).

While there is ongoing concern that recurrent hypoglyce-mic episodes might cause permanent cognitive impairments, particularly in young children (Hershey et al. 2005, 2010; Perantie et al. 2007; Northam 2001, 2009; Biessels et al. 2008; Åsvold et al. 2010; Blasetti et al. 2011), the results of long-term follow-up of DCCT patients (DCCT/EDIC 2007; Jacobson et al. 2011) are to a large extent reassuring. In 1,144 patients with type 1 diabetes (40% of whom suffered at least one episode of hypoglycemic coma or seizure) followed for a mean of 18 years, hypoglycemia was not associated with a decline in any cognitive domain. Nonetheless, in children with type 1 diabetes, repeated severe hypoglycemia, particularly that beginning before the age of 4–5 years, has been associated with impaired spatial long-term memory performance (Hershey et al. 2005), lower intel-ligence quotient scores (Northam et al. 2001, 2009) and impaired cognitive performance (Blasetti et al. 2011). It has also been associated with smaller left superior temporal gray matter volumes (Perantie et al. 2007) or decreases in occipital/parietal white matter volume (Perantie et al. 2011), larger hippocampal volumes (Hershey 2010), and volume reduction in the thalamus (Northam et al. 2009), as measured with magnetic resonance imaging. Thus, with the patient who dies from hypoglycemia aside, recurrent hypoglycemia does not appear to cause cogni-tive impairment in young to middle-aged adults with type 1 diabetes (DCCT/EDIC 2007; Jacobson et al. 2011). However, not only did the DCCT/EDIC population not include chil-dren, it also did not include elderly persons. In the Fremantle study of patients with type 2 diabetes >70 years of age at baseline, there was no relationship between a history of severe hypoglycemia and cognitive decline during follow-up (Bruce et al. 2009). However, only 205 patients were followed and only 33 experienced cognitive decline over a mean of 1.6 years. In contrast, a retrospective analysis of data from 16,667 patients with type 2 diabetes and a mean age of 65 years disclosed a graded relationship between episodes of severe hypoglycemia and dementia risk (Whitmer et al. 2009). The hazard ratios were 1.3, 1.8, and 1.9 for one, two, or three or more episodes of severe hypoglycemia, respectively. Furthermore, a population-based study disclosed an association between a self-reported history of severe hypoglycemia and poorer late-life cognitive ability in people with type 2 diabetes (Aung et al. 2012).

At the very least, an episode of hypoglycemia is a nuisance and a distraction. Hypoglycemia can be embarrassing and lead to social ostracism or employment discrimination. It can be mistaken for alcohol intoxication or illicit drug use. The resulting aberrant behavior and impaired judgment can lead to offensive acts, and altered psychomotor functions can cause impaired performance of physical tasks (such as driving). Indeed, drivers with both type 1 and insulin-treated type-2 diabetes acknowledge some unsafe driving practices during hypoglycemia (Bell et al. 2010). In type 1 diabetes, hypoglycemia-related driving mishaps have been associated with a history of severe hypoglycemia (Cox et al. 2009) as well as with a lower A1C level and a history of severe hypoglycemia (Redelmeier et al. 2009). The psychological morbidity of iatrogenic hypoglycemia includes fear of an episode (which can be a barrier to glycemic control), guilt about that fear, higher levels of anxiety, and lower levels of overall happiness (Jacobsen 1996). Fear of hypoglycemia is common, and associated with the experience of severe hypoglycemia (Beléndez and Hernández-Mijares 2009).

Mortality

The vast majority of episodes of hypoglycemia, including severe episodes that cause functional brain failure—impaired cognition, aberrant behavior, even seizure or loss of consciousness—are corrected after the plasma glucose concentration is raised. Notably, however, a self-report of severe hypoglycemia was found to be associated with a 3.6-fold higher risk of death over five years with no apparent difference in morbidity at baseline (McCoy et al. 2012). Prolonged, profound hypoglycemia can cause brain death, but that is very rare and most fatal episodes are the result of other mechanisms, presumably cardiac arrhythmias (Cryer 2007; Frier et al. 2011; Cryer 2011c).

Older estimates were that 2 to 4% of people with type 1 diabetes died from hypoglycemia (Deckert et al. 1978; Tunbridge 1981; Laing et al. 1999). More recent reports in type 1 diabetes include hypoglycemic mortality rates of 4% (Patterson et al. 2007), 6% (DCCT/EDIC 2007), 7% (Feltbower et al. 2008), and 10% (Skrivarhaug et al. 2006). Whatever the precise frequency, there is clearly an iatrogenic mortality rate in type 1 diabetes. An example, documented with continuous subcutaneous glucose monitoring, has been reported (Figure 1.1) (Tanenberg et al. 2010).

Iatrogenic hypoglycemia mortality rates in type 2 diabetes are as yet unknown. It has been reported that up to 10% of patients with severe sulfonylurea-induced hypoglycemia die (Ferner and Neil 1988; Gerich 1989; Holstein and Egberts 2003). Thus, there is reason to be concerned about the possibility of hypoglycemia-induced mortality in type 2 diabetes.

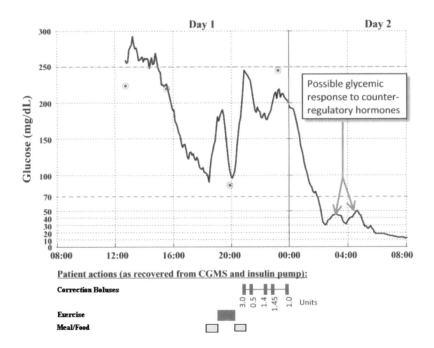

Figure 1.1. Continuous subcutaneous glucose monitoring data from a patient with type 1 diabetes the afternoon, evening, and night before he was found dead in bed. The self plasma glucose monitoring values obtained by the patient are shown by the four circles. The times of insulin boluses, exercise, and food ingestion are also shown. From Tanenberg, et al. 2010, with permission from the American Association of Clinical Endocrinologists.

Indeed, an association between hypoglycemic episodes and acute cardiovascular events in type 2 diabetes has been reported (Johnston et al. 2011) and a Danish survey disclosed increased cardiovascular and all-cause mortality in patients treated with glimepiride, glyburide (glibenclamide), glipizide, or tolbutamide compared with those treated with metformin (Schramm et al. 2011).

Increased mortality has been reported in randomized controlled trials during more intensive compared with less intensive glucose-lowering therapy in patients with type 2 diabetes (Action to Control Cardiovascular Risk in Diabetes [ACCORD] Study Group 2008) and in intensive care unit patients with hyperglycemia (The normoglycemia in Intensive Care Evaluation—Survival Using Glucose Algorithm Regulation [NICE–SUGAR] Study Investigators 2009). Given the association between hypoglycemia and mortality in these and other studies in type 2 diabetes (ADVANCE 2008; Duckworth et al. VADT 2009) and the fact that hypoglycemia can be fatal (Cryer 2007, 2011c; Lee et al. 2004; Adler et al. 2009; Nordin 2010; Frier et al. 2011), it is reasonable to suspect that iatrogenic hypoglycemia was the cause of excess mortality.

Excess mortality during intensive glycemic therapy of T2DM in ACCORD (2008) could have been the result of chance, a nonglycemic effect of some aspect of the intensive therapy regimen such as weight gain or a side-effect of one or more of the drugs administered (although none was identified), or hypoglycemia (Riddle et al. 2010; Lachin 2010; Riddle 2010). Contrary conclusions (Miller et al. 2010; Bonds et al. 2010; ACCORD 2011) notwithstanding, it is not possible to conclude with certainty whether hypoglycemia was or was not the cause of excess mortality since plasma glucose concentrations at the times of death in each of the patients in both the intensive and the conventional therapy groups are not known. However, the treatment goal of intensive therapy in ACCORD was a very aggressive A1C of <6%—with monthly addition of a new medication or drug dosage intensification if the A1C was >5.9% or if plasma glucose goals were not being met. Notably, mortality in the intensive therapy group was directly related to the A1C level (Riddle et al. 2010). Thus, it appears that rather than attaining an A1C of <6%, striving for that A1C but failing to achieve it resulted in excess mortality in ACCORD (Skyler 2010). It is not known what drugs were being added or having their dosages intensified at the times of death of these patients, but it seems likely at that point in the trial that it was often an increase in the dose of an insulin secretagogue or of insulin. Insulin excess causes death by causing hypoglycemia. The findings of similar all-cause mortality and severe hypoglycemia rates in the two treatment groups after the transition to less intensive glucose-lowering therapy in all patients (ACCORD 2011) further indicates that some aspect of intensive therapy, such as hypoglycemia, was the cause of the excessive mortality during earlier intensive glycemic therapy.

It is conceivable that hypoglycemia was a marker of more lethal underlying disease rather than the cause of mortality in ACCORD, ADVANCE, and VADT (e.g., Zoungas et al. 2010), although it is also conceivable that hypoglycemia might be likely to trigger a fatal arrhythmia in the setting of a potentially lethal disorder such as ischemic heart disease and it is not clear how an underlying lethal disease would cause severe hypoglycemia, the putative marker. However, McCoy et al. (2012) found no difference in the Charlson comorbidity index but a more than 3-fold increased mortality after five years in patients with diabetes who reported severe hypoglycemia, compared with those who reported no or mild hypoglycemia, at baseline. Furthermore, the finding of excess mortality in patients with type 2 diabetes with A1C levels in the lower, as well as the higher, range (Currie et al. 2010; Colayco et al. 2011; Huang 2011) would seem to imply a direct effect of recurrent hypoglycemia. In the UK General Practice Research Database (Currie et al. 2010) the risk of mortality in patients with T2DM and A1C levels in the lower (as well as in the higher) deciles was increased in those treated with a sulfonylurea and, to a greater extent, in those treated with insulin. (That finding was not confirmed statistically in data from the Swedish National Diabetes Register (NDR) [Eeg-Olofsson et al. 2010] but the oral agent- and insulin treated sample sizes were approximately one-quarter and one-third of those in the report of Currie and colleagues [2011].) In the data of Colayco et al. (2010), the risk of a cardiovascular event (nonfatal myocardial infarction or stroke or cardiovascular death) was increased in patients with T2DM and low (as well as high) A1C levels and in those treated with a sulfonylurea or with insulin—drugs that can cause hypoglycemia—but not in those treated with metformin. An association between A1C levels <6% and mortality in older patients with type 2 diabetes (Huang et al. 2011) and between lower, as well as higher, A1C levels and all-cause mortality in patients with diabetes and stage 3–4 chronic kidney disease (Shurraw et al. 2011; Ricks et al. 2012) has also been reported. An epidemiological association of increased mortality of initially nondiabetic individuals with low A1C levels (Selvin et al. 2010) was not confirmed (Pfister et al. 2011). In the latter data set the hazard ratio for all-cause mortality was virtually constant across the low A1C range and only began to increase when the A1C was 5.5% to 6.0% in initially nondiabetic individuals.

The clinical implication of these data is that overly aggressive glucose-lowering therapy may cause excess mortality in diabetes, i.e., that there is a limit to the degree of glycemic control that can be maintained safely with currently available methods.

The possible mechanisms of lethal hypoglycemia-induced

ventricular arrhythmias (Lee et al. 2004; Adler et al. 2009; Laitenen et al. 2008; Nordin 2010; Frier et al. 2011; Cryer 2011c) are discussed in Chapter 3. The relevance of these findings to glycemic goals and the extent to which technological advances might permit lower glycemic goals in the future are discussed in Chapter 6.

SUMMARY

Hypoglycemia is a problem for many people with diabetes that has not been solved. It is fundamentally iatrogenic, the result of therapeutic hyperinsulinemia. However, because of the effectiveness of normal defenses against falling plasma glucose concentrations (Chapter 2), hypoglycemia is relatively uncommon early in the course of type 2 diabetes (and is uncommon very early—the "honeymoon" period—in type 1 diabetes). However, hypoglycemia becomes more common over time as those defenses become compromised (Chapter 3). Understanding the latter pathophysiology leads to insight into the risk factors for (Chapter 4), definition and classification of (Chapter 5), and prevention or treatment of (Chapter 6) iatrogenic hypoglycemia in diabetes.

Chapter 2.
The Physiology of Glucose Counterregulation

HYPOGLYCEMIA AND THE BRAIN

Glucose is an obligate oxidative fuel for the brain under physiological conditions (Clarke and Sokoloff 1994; Cryer 2007, 2008, 2010, 2011a). Although the adult human brain constitutes only ~2% of body weight, it accounts for ~25% of whole-body glucose utilization. Thus, survival of the brain, and therefore the individual, requires a virtually continuous supply of glucose to the brain.

Neurons normally oxidize lactate as well as glucose, but that is largely lactate derived from glucose within the brain—mostly glucose transported from the circulation into the brain but partly that derived from glycogen in astrocytes (Itoh et al. 2003; Hyder et al. 2006; Magistretti 2006). The brain can use fuels other than glucose from the circulation if their circulating levels rise high enough to enter the brain in quantity. A commonly cited example is ketone bodies that are elevated during prolonged fasting (Owen et al. 1969) and during breast feeding in infants (Nehlig 2004). Another example is lactate that is sufficiently elevated during very vigorous exercise (Dalsgaard 2006). Nonetheless, among the potential substrates that normally circulate, including β-hydroxybutyrate and lactate, only injection of glucose has been found to rescue the brain of a hypoglycemic animal (Clarke and Sokoloff 1994; Won et al. 2012).

At elevated, physiological, or even slightly subphysiological (e.g., 65 mg/dl [3.6 mmol/l]) plasma glucose concentrations, the rate of blood-to-brain glucose transport exceeds the rate of brain glucose metabolism (Fanelli et al. 1998; Segel et al. 2001). Thus, all of the glucose required to provide oxidative fuel to the brain can be accounted for by glucose from the circulation (Wahren et al. 1999; Lubow et al. 2006). The balance of the glucose transported into the brain is either stored as (astrocytic) glycogen or transported back into the circulation.

Direct studies of human brain substrate utilization during hypoglycemia are limited. In a study of rather brief (<40 minutes) but substantial (43 mg/dl [2.4 mmol/l]) hypoglycemia in healthy humans, brain glucose uptake accounted for ~90% of brain oxygen consumption, and there was no net uptake of lactate or pyruvate, β-hydroxybutyrate, or any of nine amino acids (Wahren et al. 1999). In another study of more sustained (<120 minutes) and nearly as substantial (54 mg/dl [3.0 mmol/l]) hypoglycemia in healthy humans, brain lactate uptake increased slightly, but that accounted for no more than 25% of the calculated brain energy deficit (Lubow et al. 2006). There was no net uptake of alanine or leucine. Thus, among the potential alternative fuels that circulate, there is some evidence that the brain switches from net release to net uptake of lactate during hypoglycemia. Brain lactate uptake is directly related to the plasma lactate concentration (Boumezbeur et al. 2010) and blood-to-brain lactate transport increases when plasma lactate levels are raised to very high concentrations by vigorous exercise (Dalsgaard 2006) or by lactate infusion coupled with exercise (van Hall et al. 2009). It is thought that such lactate oxidation might support 5 to 10% of neuronal metabolic needs (Herzog et al. 2011).

Interestingly, in a study employing ^{13}C nuclear magnetic resonance spectroscopy during [^{13}C]glucose infusion in eight healthy humans, van de Ven et al. (2011) found the incorporation of glucose metabolites within the brain to be similar during euglycemia and hypoglycemia (54 mg/dl [3.0 mmol/l]); calculated tricarboxylic acid cycle rates were 0.48 ± 0.03 and 0.43 ± 0.08 μmol.g^{-1}lmin.$^{-1}$ respectively. The failure to find a significant decrease in brain oxidative metabolism during hypoglycemia might have been the result of 1) a small sample size, 2) measurement in only one region of the brain (the occipital cortex) or 3) increased oxidation of an alternative fuel such as lactate (Herzog et al. 2011), although van de Ven et al. (2011) considered the latter unlikely. Alternatively, it could be that the glycemic threshold for a decrease in brain oxidative metabolism (as opposed to that for a decrease in blood-to-brain glucose transport) is lower than the plasma glucose level of 54 mg/dl (3.0 mmol/l) studied.

At some level of hypoglycemia—perhaps <50–55 mg/dl (2.8-3.0 mmol/l), since symptoms develop in healthy humans at about that level (Schwartz et al. 1987; Mitrakou et al. 1991; Fanelli et al. 1994a)—when the rate of blood-to-brain glucose transport becomes limiting to that of brain glucose metabolism, astrocytic glycogen could be a reserve source of glucose that fuels astrocytes and (largely as lactate produced by glycolysis of glycogen-derived glucose) neurons (Öz et al. 2007). However, that reserve is limited. The brain glycogen concentration is ~1% of that in liver and 10% of that in skeletal muscle. Based on rates of brain glucose metabolism measured with [1-^{11}C] glucose and positron emission tomography in healthy humans of 0.17 μmol$\bullet$g$^{-1}\bullet$min^{-1} (Fanelli et al. 1998; Segel et al. 2001) and a brain glycogen content measured with [1-^{13}C]glucose and nuclear magnetic resonance spectroscopy in healthy humans of 3.5 μmol/g glucosyl units (Öz et al. 2007), one can calculate that glycogen in the adult human brain could support brain oxidative metabolism for ~20 minutes if brain glycogen were to become the sole source of glucose (and thus lactate). (That 20-minute oxidative reserve from glycogen calculated from human data is remarkably similar to the finding of compound action potential failure of mouse optic nerves 15.9±0.4 minutes after initial exposure to glucose-free artificial cerebrospinal fluid [Brown et al. 2005].) Even if blood-to-brain glucose transport were to account for 90% of brain glucose metabolism during mild-to-moderate hypoglycemia (Fanelli et al. 1998; Segel et al. 2001; Wahren et al. 1999; Lubow et al. 2006), the 10% supply of brain glycogen-derived glucose (and lactate) would be exhausted in ~200 minutes.

In summary, because it cannot synthesize glucose, use physiological levels of circulating non-glucose fuels effectively, or store more than 20 minutes' supply as glycogen, the brain requires a virtually continuous supply of glucose from the circulation. Because facilitated blood-to-brain glucose transport (mediated by glucose transporter1) is a direct function of the arterial plasma glucose concentration, maintenance of the plasma glucose concentration at or above the normal range is required. At low plasma glucose concentrations, functional brain failure (and, if hypoglycemia is profound and prolonged, brain death) occurs (Cryer 2007).

RESPONSES TO HYPOGLYCEMIA

Falling plasma glucose concentrations elicit a characteristic sequence of responses in humans (Schwartz et al. 1987;

Mitrakou et al. 1991; Fanelli et al. 1994a). These are shown diagrammatically in Figure 2.1 and are detailed in Table 2.1. The earliest physiological response is a decrease in insulin secretion. That occurs as plasma glucose levels decline within the physiological range. The secretion of glucose counterregulatory (plasma glucose–raising) hormones, including glucagon and epinephrine, increases as plasma glucose concentrations fall just below the postabsorptive physiological range. Lower glucose levels cause symptoms. Even lower levels cause functional brain failure (Cryer 2007). Prolonged, very low levels can cause brain death (Cryer 2007).

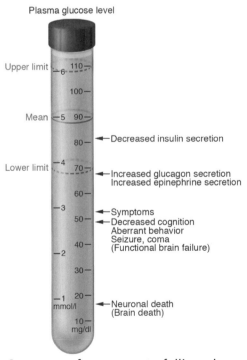

Figure 2.1. Sequence of responses to falling plasma glucose concentrations in humans. From Cryer 2007, with permission from the American Society for Clinical Investigation.

Table 2.1 Physiological Responses to Decreasing Plasma Glucose Concentrations

Response	Glycemic threshold* [mg/dl (mmol/l)]	Physiological effects	Role in prevention or correction of hypoglycemia (glucose counterregulation)
↓ Insulin	80–85 (4.4–4.7)	↑R_a (↓R_d)	Primary glucose regulatory factor, first defense against hypoglycemia
↑ Glucagon	65–70 (3.6–3.9)	↑R_a	Primary glucose counterregulatory factor, second defense against hypoglycemia
↑ Epinephrine	65–70 (3.6–3.9)	↑R_a, ↓R_c	Involved, critical when glucagon is deficient, third defense against hypoglycemia
↑ Cortisol and growth hormone	65–70 (3.6–3.9)	↑R_a, ↓R_c	Involved, not critical
Symptoms	50–55 (2.8–3.1)	↑Exogenous glucose	Prompt behavioral defense (food ingestion)
↓ Cognition	<50 (<2.8)	—	Compromises behavioral defense

*Arterialized venous, not venous, plasma glucose concentrations. R_a, rate of glucose appearance, glucose production by the liver and kidneys; R_d, rate of glucose disappearance, glucose utilization by insulin-sensitive tissues such as skeletal muscle (no direct effect on central nervous system glucose utilization); R_c rate of glucose clearance by insulin sensitive tissues.

CLINICAL MANIFESTATIONS OF HYPOGLYCEMIA

Symptoms and signs of hypoglycemia are not specific (Towler et al. 1993). Thus, hypoglycemia is documented most convincingly by Whipple's triad (Whipple 1938): symptoms, signs, or both consistent with hypoglycemia, a low reliably measured plasma glucose concentration, and resolution of those symptoms and signs after the plasma glucose level is raised (Cryer et al. 2009). A requirement for formal documentation of Whipple's triad—including a laboratory measurement of a low plasma glucose concentration—is important for the initial demonstration that a hypoglycemic disorder exists in patients without diabetes, since such disorders are rare (Cryer et al. 2009; Cryer 2011a). On the other hand, in patients with diabetes treated with insulin, a sulfonylurea, or a glinide, the likelihood that a given symptomatic episode is the result of hypoglycemia is high (Chapter 1). Ideally, such patients should always estimate their plasma glucose concentrations with a monitor when they suspect their glucose level is low. In reality, that is sometimes not practical and it is often not done. Nonetheless, it could be reasoned that the detrimental effects of brief erroneous treatment for suspected hypoglycemia are less than those of failure to treat an episode of bona fide hypoglycemia (Cryer 2007).

Symptoms

Symptoms of hypoglycemia are categorized as neuroglycopenic—those that are the direct result of brain glucose deprivation per se—and neurogenic (or autonomic)—those that are largely the result of the perception of physiological changes caused by the central nervous system (CNS)–mediated sympathoadrenal discharge triggered by hypoglycemia (Cryer 2007, 2008, 2010, 2011a; Schwartz et al. 1987; Mitrakou et al. 1991; Fanelli et al. 1994a; Towler et al. 1993; Deary et al. 1993; De Rosa and Cryer 2004) (Figure 2.1 and Table 2.1). (There is a semantic issue here. Neurogenic symptoms are initiated by glucose deprivation at peripheral and central sensors, i.e., by neuroglycopenia. However, their generation includes activation of sympathoadrenal outflow from the brain through the spinal cord to preganglionic neurons innervating the adrenal medullae and sympathetic postganglionic neurons, and they are largely sympathetic neural in origin [DeRosa and Cryer 2004].)

Neuroglycopenic manifestations of hypoglycemia include cognitive impairments, behavioral changes, and psychomotor abnormalities, and, at lower plasma glucose levels, seizure and coma—all examples of functional brain failure (Cryer 2007). Ultimately, after profound, prolonged hypoglycemia, they include brain death (Cryer 2007).

Neurogenic manifestations of hypoglycemia include both adrenergic and cholinergic symptoms (Towler et al. 1993). These are largely the result of sympathetic neural rather than adrenomedullary activation, since bilaterally adrenalectomized individuals experience typical neurogenic symptoms (DeRosa and Cryer 2004). Adrenergic symptoms—mediated largely by norepinephrine released from sympathetic postganglionic neurons but perhaps also to some extent by circulating epinephrine released from the adrenal medullae—include palpitations, tremor, and anxiety/arousal (Towler et al. 1993; DeRosa and Cryer 2004). Cholinergic symptoms—mediated largely by acetylcholine released from sympathetic postganglionic neurons—include sweating, hunger, and paresthesias (Towler et al. 1993; DeRosa and Cryer 2004). This classification is based on the effects of adrenergic and cholinergic antagonists (Towler et al. 1993). To the extent that those antagonists enter the brain, some of these symptoms (e.g., anxiety/arousal and hunger [Schultes et al. 2003]) may be mediated through central as well as peripheral mechanisms. Principal components analysis leads to a somewhat different classification of the symptoms of hypoglycemia (Deary et al. 1993; McCrimmon et al. 2003a).

Awareness of hypoglycemia is largely the result of the perception of neurogenic symptoms. It is reduced substantially by combined adrenergic and cholinergic antagonism in humans

(Towler et al. 1993). Thus, it follows that hypoglycemia unawareness in people with diabetes (Chapter 3) is largely the result of reduced sympathetic neural, rather than adrenomedullary, activation during hypoglycemia. It is true that patients endorse both neurogenic and neuroglycopenic symptoms of hypoglycemia (Cox et al. 1993), but the extent to which they interpret neuroglycopenic symptoms as indicative of hypoglycemia is unclear.

Signs

Pallor and diaphoresis (caused by adrenergic cutaneous vasoconstriction and cholinergic stimulation of sweat glands, respectively) are common signs of hypoglycemia. Heart rate and systolic blood pressure are raised, but usually not greatly. Neuroglycopenic manifestations are often observable. Transient neurological deficits sometimes occur.

SYSTEMIC GLUCOSE BALANCE

Normally, rates of glucose flux into and out of the circulation are coordinately regulated such that systemic glucose balance is maintained, hypoglycemia (as well as hyperglycemia) is prevented, and a continuous supply of glucose to the brain is assured (Cryer 2001, 2008, 2010, 2011a) (Table 2.2).

Glucose influx into the circulation is the sum of intermittent exogenous glucose delivery from ingested carbohydrates and regulated endogenous glucose production from the liver (glycogenolysis and gluconeogenesis) and the kidneys (gluconeogenesis). Glucose efflux out of the circulation is the sum of ongoing fixed glucose utilization, largely by the brain, but to a small extent by strictly glycolytic tissues such as the renal

Table 2.2. Systemic Glucose Balance

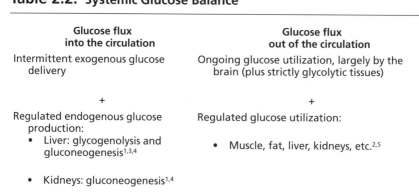

Glucose flux into the circulation	Glucose flux out of the circulation
Intermittent exogenous glucose delivery	Ongoing glucose utilization, largely by the brain (plus strictly glycolytic tissues)
+	+
Regulated endogenous glucose production: • Liver: glycogenolysis and gluconeogenesis[1,3,4] • Kidneys: gluconeogenesis[1,4]	Regulated glucose utilization: • Muscle, fat, liver, kidneys, etc.[2,5]

[1]Decreased by insulin; [2]increased by insulin; [3]increased by glucagon; [4]increased by epinephrine; [5]decreased by epinephrine.

medullae and erythrocytes, and regulated glucose utilization by insulin-sensitive tissues such as muscle, fat, liver, and kidneys among others. Because exogenous glucose delivery is intermittent and much of glucose utilization (largely that by the brain) is fixed, the plasma glucose concentration is maintained and systemic glucose balance is fine-tuned by regulated endogenous glucose production and regulated glucose utilization by non-neural tissues (Cryer 2001, 2008, 2010, 2011a; Cherrington 2001).

The liver is the major site of net endogenous glucose production but net renal glucose production has been demonstrated under some conditions, including prolonged fasting and hypoglycemia, in humans (Gerich et al. 2001; Gerich 2010). Resumption of endogenous glucose production during the anhepatic phase of human liver transplantation (Joseph et al. 2000) documented extra-hepatic glucose production, and data from a mouse model of inducible liver-specific deletion of the glucose-6-phosphatase gene provided evidence of physiologically important extra-hepatic glucose production (Mutel et al. 2011). In the latter animals fasting plasma glucose concentrations fell initially but then became similar to those in control animals after ~30 hours, a finding attributed by the authors to increased renal and intestinal glucose production.

Although an array of hormonal, neural, and substrate factors are involved, glucose production and utilization are regulated primarily by the pancreatic β-cell hormone insulin. As plasma glucose concentrations rise (e.g., after a meal), insulin secretion increases and both suppresses hepatic (and renal) glucose production and stimulates glucose utilization by muscle and fat. As plasma glucose concentrations decline (e.g., between meals), insulin secretion decreases and both increases hepatic (and renal) glucose production and decreases glucose utilization by muscle and fat. Importantly, although insulin does act on regions of the brain—to improve memory (Craft et al. 1996; Kern et al. 2001; Benedict et al. 2004, 2007), decrease appetite (Porte et al. 2005), activate parasympathetic inhibition of endogenous glucose production (Obici et al. 2002), activate hepatic glycogen synthesis (Ramnanan et al. 2011b), and modulate regional glucose metabolism (Bingham et al. 2002), among other effects (Benedict et al. 2006)—it does not stimulate blood-to-brain glucose transport (Knudsen et al. 1999; Seaquist et al. 2001).

Insulin is a potent and critical hormone. Its deficiency causes hyperglycemia (diabetes), and its excess can cause hypoglycemia (Cryer 2001, 2008, 2010, 2011a; Cherrington 2001; Cryer et al. 2009). Nonetheless, it is not the only factor involved in maintenance of systemic glucose balance. The plasma glucose-raising (glucose counterregulatory) hormones glucagon, epinephrine, cortisol, and growth hormone are also involved.

GLUCOREGULATORY FACTORS

Insulin

Insulin secretion is stimulated by glucose, amino acids, non-esterified fatty acids, β_2-adrenergic activation by catecholamines such as epinephrine, acetylcholine released from parasympathetic nerves, glucagon-like peptide-1, and glucose-dependent insulinotropic polypeptide; it is inhibited by low glucose, α_2-adrenergic activation by catecholamines such as norepinephrine released from sympathetic nerves, and somatostatin. Insulin secretion is very sensitive to fluctuations in the plasma glucose concentration within the physiological range (Cryer 2001, 2008, 2010, 2011a; Cherrington 2001; Heller and Cryer 1991a) (Table 2.1).

Insulin is secreted from pancreatic islet β-cells into the hepatic portal vein. Approximately 50% is extracted by the liver (Cherrington 2001). Insulin secretion can be quantified by measurements of the plasma concentrations of C-peptide, the peptide cleaved from proinsulin to produce insulin (Eaton et al. 1980; Polonsky et al. 1986). C-peptide is co-secreted with insulin but not cleared by the liver. Insulin secretion so calculated virtually ceases during hypoglycemia in humans (Heller and Cryer 1991a).

The physiology of insulin action has been reviewed (Ferrannini 2012). Insulin suppresses hepatic glycogenolysis rapidly and hepatic (and renal) gluconeogenesis more gradually and thus suppresses endogenous glucose production (Cryer 2001, 2008, 2010, 2011a; Cherrington 2001; Edgerton et al. 2006). Basal insulin levels restrain glucose production in the postabsorptive state, and increased insulin levels suppress glucose production and stimulate glucose utilization in the postprandial state. The actions of insulin to suppress glucose production are both direct (via hepatic and renal insulin receptors) and indirect (Cryer 2001, 2008, 2010, 2011a; Cherrington 2001; Obici et al. 2002; Edgerton et al. 2006, 2011; Bergman 2007). The hormone acts indirectly by inhibition of lipolysis, suppression of glucagon secretion, limitation of gluconeogenic precursor (e.g., lactate, amino acids, glycerol) flux from muscle and fat to the liver (and kidneys), and CNS-mediated activation of parasympathetic outflow.

Conversely, a decrease in insulin, as during decreasing plasma glucose concentrations and hypoglycemia, causes an increase in hepatic (and renal) glucose production, again initially an increase in hepatic glycogenolysis, and virtual cessation of glucose utilization by insulin-sensitive tissues (Cryer 2001, 2008, 2010, 2011a; Cherrington 2001; Heller and Cryer 1991a). As discussed later in this chapter, a decrease in insulin is the first physiological defense against hypoglycemia (Cryer 2001, 2008).

Glucagon

Glucagon secretion is stimulated by low glucose, amino acids, β_2-adrenergic activation by catecholamines such as epinephrine and norepinephrine, acetylcholine released from parasympathetic nerves, and glucose-dependent insulinotropic polypeptide; it is inhibited by high glucose, insulin, nonesterified fatty acids, somatostatin, and glucagon-like peptide-1 (Cryer 2001, 2008, 2010, 2011a; Cherrington 2001). Whereas it is less sensitive to decreasing glucose levels than insulin secretion, glucagon secretion increases as plasma glucose concentrations fall just below the physiological range (Schwartz et al. 1987; Mitrakou et al. 1991; Fanelli et al. 1994a) (Table 2.1).

A decrease in β-cell insulin secretion normally stimulates glucagon secretion during hypoglycemia (Maruyama et al. 1984; Samols et al. 1988; Banarer et al. 2002; Raju and Cryer 2005; Gosmanov et al. 2005; Israelian et al. 2005; Cooperberg and Cryer 2009, 2010a). The regulation of glucagon secretion by nutrients, hormones, neurotransmitters, and drugs is complex and incompletely understood (Cooperberg and Cryer 2009, 2010a). It involves direct signaling of α-cells (Walker et al. 2011), indirect intra-islet signaling of α-cells by β-cell secretory products including insulin (Cooperberg and Cryer 2010a) and the δ-cell secretory product somatostatin (Hauge-Evans et al. 2009), and indirect extra-islet signaling by the autonomic nervous system (Taborsky et al. 1998; Marty et al. 2007) and by gut incretins (Holst et al. 2007). Among the intra-islet factors, β-cell secretion appears to play an important role since selective destruction of β-cells in T1DM results in loss of the glucagon secretory response to hypoglycemia (Gerich et al. 1973) and partial reduction of β-cell mass in minipigs results in impaired postprandial suppression of glucagon secretion (Meier et al. 2006). Glucagon secretion is not critically dependent on extra-islet signaling. Hypoglycemia increases glucagon secretion from the denervated (transplanted) human pancreas (Diem et al. 1990) and the denervated dog pancreas (Sherck et al. 2001), as well as in the spinal cord-transected human (Palmer et al. 1976), and the glucagon response is quantitatively normal. Furthermore, low glucose increases glucagon secretion from the perfused rodent pancreas (Gerich et al. 1974) and perifused rodent and human islets (Walker et al. 2011), i.e., in the absence of neural and gut factors. There is evidence that insulin restrains glucagon secretion partially through central actions as well as through direct α-cell actions (Paranjape et al. 2010). But, again, glucagon secretion is not critically dependent on extra-islet signaling. The evidence that insulin reciprocally regulates glucagon secretion has been reviewed (Cryer 2012).

Glucagon is secreted from pancreatic islet α-cells into the hepatic portal vein. Approximately 25% is extracted by the liver (Cherrington 2001). The hormone generally is thought to act only on the liver where it stimulates glucose production (Ramnanan et al. 2011a); however, it is lipolytic in high doses. The absence of a marker of glucagon secretion (analogous to C-peptide for insulin secretion) complicates the assessment of glucagon secretion in humans. Furthermore, available glucagon immunoassays measure species in addition to biologically active 3,500-Dalton glucagon, although changes in measured glucagon levels are thought to reflect changes in biologically active glucagon (Cherrington 2001). In addition, because insulin suppresses glucagon secretion, the glucagon responses to hypoglycemia measured during contemporary hyperinsulinemic-hypoglycemic clamps are much less robust than the responses measured during hypoglycemia induced by an intravenous bolus injection of insulin.

Glucagon rapidly stimulates hepatic (but not renal) glucose production, largely by stimulating glycogenolysis (Cryer 2001, 2008, 2010; Cherrington 2001; Ramnanan et al. 2011a). The increase in glucose production and the plasma glucose concentration are transient, in part because of increased insulin secretion and the suppressive effect of hyperglycemia on glucose production (Cherrington 2001). Glucagon also stimulates hepatic gluconeogenesis when gluconeogenic precursors are abundant, as they are when epinephrine levels are also elevated (Gustavson et al. 2003). The hepatic glycogenolytic response to glucagon is enhanced by nearly 3-fold during insulin-induced hypoglycemia (Rivera et al. 2010). The extent to which that increased sensitivity to glucagon over insulin is the result of a synergistic interaction between glucagon and other glucose-raising systems, such as the sympathoadrenal system, activated by hypoglycemia, by hypoglycemia per se, or both is not known.

Glucagon, in concert with insulin, supports the postabsorptive plasma glucose concentration in humans (Cherrington 2001; Breckenridge et al. 2007; Cooperberg and Cryer 2010b). Indeed, glucagon likely plays a role in the pathogenesis of hyperglycemia in diabetes (Unger and Orci 1975; Lee et al. 2011; Edgerton and Cherrington 2011; Cryer 2012). As discussed later in this chapter, an increase in glucagon is the second physiological defense against hypoglycemia (Cryer 2001, 2008).

Epinephrine and the sympathoadrenal system

The autonomic nervous system includes the sympathetic nervous system and the adrenal medullae, collectively termed the sympathoadrenal system, and the parasympathetic nervous system. All three components are involved in metabolic regulation, including glucoregulation (Cryer 2001, 2008, 2010, 2011a): sympathoadrenal activation raises plasma glucose concentrations and parasympathetic activation tends to lower plasma glucose concentrations. Postganglionic sympathetic neurons release norepinephrine or acetylcholine, and postganglionic parasympathetic neurons release acetylcholine, within innervated tissues. Whereas some extra-adrenal chromaffin cells persist into adult life, the major residual clusters of chromaffin cells comprise the adrenal medullae, which are virtually the sole source of the circulating hormone epinephrine (Cryer 2001, 2008, 2010, 2011a; DeRosa and Cryer 2004). The anatomical relationship between the adrenal medullae and the adrenal cortices is important physiologically since a portal venous system provides cortisol from the cortex to the medulla, where the enzyme that catalyzes the conversion of norepinephrine to epinephrine (phenylethanolamine-N-methyltransferase) is cortisol induced (Wurtman and Axelrod 1965; Wurtman 2002). Thus, adrenocortical cortisol deficiency results in adrenomedullary epinephrine deficiency (Wurtman 2002), including a markedly reduced plasma epinephrine response to hypoglycemia in humans (Davis et al. 1997a).

Unlike insulin and glucagon secretion, which are regulated primarily by changes in glucose concentrations within the pancreatic islets and only secondarily by autonomic mechanisms, sympathoadrenal activity, including epinephrine secretion, is regulated within the CNS (Cryer 2001, 2008). For example, subphysiological plasma glucose concentrations, sensed in the periphery (e.g., in the portal vein) and in the CNS (Sherwin 2008; Levin et al. 2008; McCrimmon and Sherwin 2010; Watts and Donovan 2010; Levin et al. 2011), trigger a centrally mediated sympathoadrenal discharge—the magnitude of which is a function of the nadir glucose concentration—resulting in an increase in circulating epinephrine and norepinephrine. The epinephrine response is derived almost exclusively from the adrenal medullae (DeRosa and Cryer 2004). Whereas circulating norepinephrine is largely derived from sympathetic nerves under resting and many stimulated (e.g., exercise) conditions (Goldstein and Kopin 2008), the increment in plasma norepinephrine during hypoglycemia is largely derived from the adrenal medullae (DeRosa and Cryer 2004).

The biochemistry and the integrated physiology of the human sympathoadrenal system have been reviewed in detail (Eisenhofer et al. 2004). Epinephrine and norepinephrine are released from adrenomedullary chromaffin cells into the circulation; as such, these catecholamines function as classical hormones (Cryer 2001, 2008, 2010, 2011a). In addition, norepinephrine is released from axon terminals of sympathetic postganglionic neurons into synaptic clefts in direct relationship to adrenergic receptors on target cells and functions as a neurotransmitter (Cryer 2001, 2008, 2010, 2011a). Most of the neurally released norepinephrine is recaptured into axon terminals (or is metabolized locally); perhaps only 10% enters the circulation. Most metabolism of catecholamines occurs in the cytoplasm of the cells in which the amines are produced as a result of leakage from storage vesicles into the cytoplasm or during transit through the cytoplasm after reuptake from the extracellular space (Eisenhofer et al. 2004). Sympathetic postganglionic neurons largely express the degradative enzyme monoamine oxidase and therefore produce deaminated metabolites of norepinephrine (e.g., 3,4-dihydroxyphenylglycol). However, adrenomedullary chromaffin cells also express the enzyme catechol-O-methyltransferase and produce primarily the 3-O-methyl metabolites of epinephrine and norepinephrine, metanephrine and normetanephrine. In humans, >90% of circulating metanephrine, and ~33% of circulating normetanephrine, are derived from the adrenal medullae (Eisenhofer et al. 2004). Thus, stimulated plasma metanephrine concentrations can be conceptualized as a measure of the adrenomedullary epinephrine secretory capacity.

Measurement of the plasma epinephrine concentration provides a useful index of adrenomedullary activity (DeRosa and Cryer 2004), although, like that of other hormones, it represents the balance between secretion and clearance. The evaluation of sympathetic neural activity is more problematic.

Although circulating norepinephrine is largely derived from adrenergic sympathetic postganglionic neurons under resting and many stimulated conditions (Goldstein and Kopin 2008), the increase in plasma norepinephrine concentrations during hypoglycemia is largely derived from the adrenal medulla (DeRosa and Cryer 2004). Furthermore, even under the appropriate conditions, circulating norepinephrine represents only a small fraction of that released from sympathetic nerves and is the net result of differentiated regional nerve firing. Isotope dilution estimates of systemic and regional norepinephrine spillover have been used to overcome these shortcomings (Eisenhofer 2005; Paramore et al. 1998) and have documented sympathetic neural responses to hypoglycemia, although the fundamental assumptions of the method have been questioned (Christensen and Norsk 2005). Microneurography measures muscle sympathetic nerve activity directly and has documented an increase in this nerve activity during hypoglycemia (Vallbo et al. 2004; Fagius 2003). However, the method is operator dependent, time-consuming, and demanding for the subject; does not allow movement by the subject; is not practical in the presence of autonomic neuropathy; and measures only one aspect of sympathetic nerve activity in only one region of the body (typically the lower extremity). Another approach is measurement of the extracellular norepinephrine concentration by microdialysis (Bruce et al. 2002; Maggs et al. 1997). That method has been used to document norepinephrine release in skeletal muscle and fat during hypoglycemia (Maggs et al. 1997). It requires careful calibration and is applicable to limited regions of the body. Finally, as noted earlier, adrenergic and cholinergic symptoms (Towler et al. 1993) reflect the sympathetic neural response to hypoglycemia (DeRosa and Cryer 2004).

Like glucagon, epinephrine rapidly stimulates hepatic gly-cogenolysis; it stimulates hepatic gluconeogenesis more prominently than glucagon (Gustavson et al. 2003). Unlike glucagon, epinephrine also stimulates renal gluconeogenesis and glucose production (Gerich 2010), limits glucose clearance by insulin-sensitive tissues such as muscle, mobilizes gluconeogenic precursors from muscle (lactate, amino acids) and fat (glycerol) to the liver and kidneys, and suppresses insulin secretion (Cryer 2001, 2008, 2010, 2011a; Gustavson et al. 2003; Rizza et al. 1980; Berk et al. 1985).

The mechanisms of the plasma glucose–raising effect of epinephrine, summarized in Figure 2.2, are complex (Cryer 1993, 2001). They involve both direct (on the liver and kidneys) and indirect (other hormone- or substrate-mediated) actions, include both stimulation of glucose production and limitation of glucose utilization, and are mediated through both β- and α-adrenergic receptors. Whereas many of the actions of the hormone involve β_2-adrenergic receptors (Figure 2.2), β_2-adrenergic activation alone has little plasma glucose–raising effect in healthy individuals because it also stimulates insulin secretion. Thus, α_2-adrenergic limitation of insulin secretion is normally an important aspect of the glycemic effect of epinephrine. Nonetheless, there is normally a small increase in insulin secretion—in response to β_2-adrenergic β-cell stimulation, rising plasma glucose concentrations, or both—over time (Berk et al. 1985). That, too, is a critical glucoregulatory event because it limits the magnitude of the glycemic response. The glycemic response to epinephrine is increased substantially when insulin secretion is held constant pharmacologically in healthy individuals and in patients with type 1 diabetes who cannot increase insulin secretion (Berk et al.

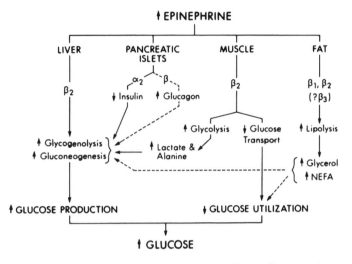

Figure 2.2. Mechanisms of the hyperglycemic effect of epinephrine. The α and β symbols refer to α-adrenergic and β-adrenergic receptors. From Cryer 1993, with permission from the American Diabetes Association.

1985). As discussed later in this chapter, an increase in epinephrine is the third defense against hypoglycemia.

Similar mechanisms are thought to be involved in the glycemic response to sympathetic neural norepinephrine release (Cryer 2001, 2008, 2010, 2011a). The adrenergic and cholinergic neurogenic symptoms caused by the intense sympathoadrenal response to frank hypoglycemia prompt awareness of hypoglycemia (Towler et al. 1993; DeRosa and Cryer 2004). As discussed later in this chapter, that awareness prompts the behavioral defense against hypoglycemia, ingestion of carbohydrates.

Cortisol and growth hormone

The plasma glucose–raising actions of glucagon and epinephrine occur within minutes (Cryer 2001, 2008; Cherrington

2001). In contrast, those of cortisol (Rizza et al. 1982) and growth hormone (MacGorman et al. 1981) (both of which support glucose production and limit glucose clearance) are delayed for several hours. Importantly, none of these hormones (glucagon, epinephrine, cortisol, or growth hormone) alters glucose transport across the blood-brain barrier.

GLUCOSE COUNTERREGULATION: THE PREVENTION AND CORRECTION OF HYPOGLYCEMIA

Physiological defenses

As reviewed in detail (Cryer 2001), there are three principles for the physiological prevention or correction of hypoglycemia (Garber et al. 1976; Clarke et al. 1979; Gerich et al. 1979; Rizza et al. 1979) (Table 2.3). First, the prevention and correction of hypoglycemia are the result of both waning of insulin and activation of glucose counterregulatory (plasma glucose–raising) systems. They are not due solely to waning of insulin. After intravenous insulin injection, the changes in glucose kinetics that ultimately restore euglycemia—an increase in insulin-suppressed glucose production and a decrease in insulin-stimulated glucose utilization—begin while plasma insulin concentrations are still 10-fold above baseline and in temporal relation to increments in the plasma levels of counterregulatory hormones (Garber et al. 1976; Clarke et al. 1979). Similarly, the changes in glucose kinetics that limit the hypoglycemic response to prolonged hyperinsulinemia occur despite sustained hyperinsulinemia (De Feo et al. 1986). In addition, hypoinsulinemia is not critical to recovery from hypoglycemia (Heller and Cryer

1991a). Furthermore, when insulin levels are held constant, interruption of the secretion or actions of glucose counterregulatory factors impairs the prevention or correction of hypoglycemia (see following). Second, whereas insulin is the dominant plasma glucose–lowering factor, there are redundant glucose counterregulatory factors (Gerich et al. 1979; Rizza et al. 1979). These collectively constitute a fail-safe system that prevents or minimizes failure of the glucose counterregulatory process upon failure of one, or perhaps more, of its components. Third, there is a hierarchy among the redundant glucoregulatory factors, i.e., a ranked series of counterregulatory factors, some more critical to the effectiveness of the fail-safe system than others, that act in concert with decrements in insulin to prevent or correct hypoglycemia (Gerich et al. 1979; Rizza et al. 1979). Several aspects of this physiology are also shown in Table 2.1. Studies of its mechanisms in humans are summarized in Figure 2.3 (Cryer 1981) and Figure 2.4 (Gerich 1988).

In defense against falling plasma glucose concentrations, decrements in insulin are fundamentally important. Insulin secretion virtually ceases during hypoglycemia and increments

---

Table 2.3. Principles of Glucose Counterregulation in Humans

1. The prevention and correction of hypoglycemia are the result of both waning of insulin and activation of glucose counterregulatory systems. They are not due solely to waning of insulin.

2. Whereas insulin is the dominant plasma glucose–lowering factor, there are redundant glucose counterregulatory factors. Those include other hormones as well as substrates and perhaps neural factors. These collectively constitute a fail-safe system.

3. There is a hierarchy among the glucoregulatory factors. Decrements in insulin, increments in glucagon, and, absent the latter, increments in epinephrine stand high in that hierarchy.

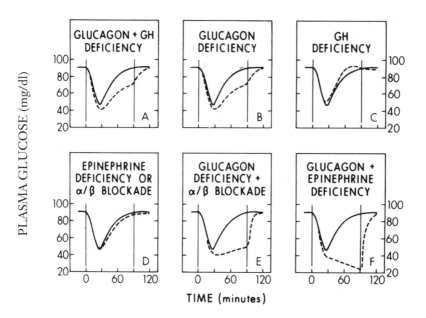

Figure 2.3. Summary of studies of the mechanisms of recovery from short-term hypoglycemia, induced by intravenous insulin injection at time 0 minutes, in humans. Interventions were started at time 0 minutes and stopped at time 90 minutes (i.e., between the vertical lines in each panel). Plasma glucose curves in control studies are indicated by the solid lines (the same in all panels), and plasma glucose curves under the indicated conditions are shown by the dashed lines. GH, growth hormone. From Cryer 1981, with permission from the American Diabetes Association.

in insulin from suppressed levels impair recovery from hypoglycemia in a dose-related fashion (Heller and Cryer 1991a). An increase in insulin secretion is the first, and for practical purposes the only, defense against rising plasma glucose concentrations; loss of β-cell insulin secretion causes hyperglycemia (diabetes mellitus) and is fatal if insulin is not replaced. Conversely, a decrease in insulin secretion is the first, and arguably the most important, defense against falling plasma glucose

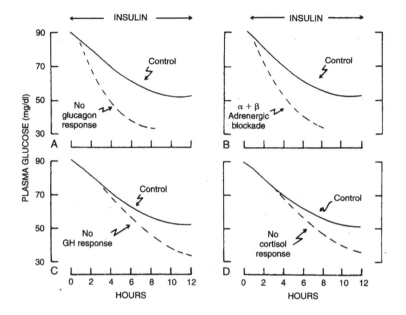

Figure 2.4. Summary of studies of the mechanisms of defense against prolonged insulin-induced hypoglycemia in humans. Plasma glucose curves in control studies are indicated by the solid lines (the same in all panels), and plasma glucose curves under the indicated conditions are shown by the dashed lines. From Gerich 1988, with permission from the American Diabetes Association.

concentrations. But, it is not the only defense. Glucose counterregulatory systems can prevent or correct hypoglycemia despite moderate hyperinsulinemia.

Among the glucose counterregulatory factors, glucagon plays a primary role (Gerich et al. 1979; Rizza et al. 1979). Albeit demonstrably involved, epinephrine is not normally critical. But, it becomes critical when glucagon is deficient. Isolated deficiency of the glucagon response (De Feo et al. 1991a) or of epinephrine actions (De Feo et al. 1991b) results in lower nadir plasma glucose concentrations early in the course of prolonged hypoglycemia. These data document that both glucagon and epinephrine are involved in defense against hyperinsulinemia. They do not address the relative roles of glucagon or epinephrine in the prevention or correction of hypoglycemia. Suppression of glucagon secretion (with somatostatin) impairs, but does not prevent, recovery from short-term hypoglycemia (Gerich et al. 1979; Rizza et al. 1979). That effect is reversed by glucagon, but not by growth hormone, replacement. In contrast, neither pharmacological adrenergic blockade nor epinephrine deficiency (bilateral adrenalectomy) impairs recovery from short-term hypoglycemia. However, progressive hypoglycemia develops when both glucagon and epinephrine are deficient. These data indicate that glucagon is involved in the correction of hypoglycemia, whereas epinephrine is not critical when glucagon secretion is intact. However, epinephrine becomes critical when glucagon secretion is deficient. Suppression of glucagon secretion lowers plasma glucose concentrations after an overnight fast (Breckenridge et al. 2007; Rosen et al. 1984; Cooperberg and Cryer 2010b), during a prolonged fast (Boyle et al. 1989), late after glucose ingestion (Tse et al. 1983a, 1983b), and during moderate exercise (Hirsch et al. 1991; Marker et al. 1991). In contrast, with the exception of a small effect during exercise, neither pharmacological adrenergic blockade nor epinephrine deficiency lowers plasma glucose concentrations under any of these conditions (Rosen et al. 1984; Boyle et al. 1989; Tse et al. 1983a, 1983b; Hirsch et al. 1991; Marker et al. 1991). However, combined glucagon deficiency and adrenergic blockade (or epinephrine deficiency) results in progressive hypoglycemia under all four conditions (Rosen et al. 1984; Boyle et al. 1989; Tse et al. 1983a, 1983b; Hirsch et al. 1991; Marker et al. 1991). These data further indicate that glucagon plays a role in the prevention and correction of hypoglycemia under diverse physiological conditions, whereas epinephrine is not critical when glucagon secretion is intact. However, epinephrine becomes critical to the prevention or correction of hypoglycemia under diverse conditions when glucagon secretion is deficient. The role of glucagon in the pathogenesis of hypoglycemia (and hyperglycemia) in diabetes has been reviewed (Cryer 2012).

Growth hormone and cortisol stand lower in the hierarchy of physiological glucose counterregulatory factors than insulin, glucagon, and epinephrine (De Feo et al. 1989a, 1989b; Boyle and Cryer 1991). Both growth hormone (De Feo et al. 1989a) and cortisol (De Feo et al. 1989b) are involved in defense against prolonged hypoglycemia, but neither is critical to the correction of even prolonged hypoglycemia or the prevention of hypoglycemia after an overnight fast (Boyle and Cryer 1991).

There is evidence that glucose autoregulation—an increase in endogenous glucose production independent of hormonal and neural regulatory signals—is involved in glucose counterregulation, albeit only during severe hypoglycemia (Bolli et al. 1985), and that nonesterified fatty acids mediate, at least in part, the glucose counterregulatory actions of epinephrine (Fanelli et al. 1992).

There is no clear evidence that efferent neural mechanisms normally play an important role in physiological glucose counterregulation. However, sympathoadrenal activation plays a key role in the behavioral defense against developing hypoglycemia.

Behavioral defense

If the physiological defenses fail to reverse falling plasma glucose concentrations, lower plasma glucose levels trigger a more intense sympathoadrenal response, which causes symptoms (Towler et al. 1993; DeRosa and Cryer 2004) that allow the individual to recognize hypoglycemia. Again, the neurogenic symptoms of hypoglycemia are largely the result of sympathetic neural, rather than adrenomedullary, activation (De Rosa and Cryer 2004). That awareness of hypoglycemia prompts the behavioral defense against hypoglycemia, ingestion of carbohydrates.

INTEGRATED PHYSIOLOGY OF GLUCOSE COUNTERREGULATION

The integrated physiology of glucose counterregulation—the mechanisms that normally prevent or rapidly correct hypoglycemia in humans (Cryer 2001)—is summarized in Figure 2.5 (Cryer 2006b). The first defense against falling plasma glucose concentrations is a decrease in pancreatic β-cell insulin secretion. The second defense is an increase in pancreatic α-cell glucagon secretion. The third defense, which becomes critical when glucagon is deficient, is an increase in adrenomedullary epinephrine secretion. If these three physiological defenses fail to abort the episode, lower plasma glucose levels trigger a more intense sympathoadrenal (sympathetic neural as well as adrenomedullary) response that causes symptoms and thus awareness of hypoglycemia that prompts the behavioral defense.

The mechanisms of the normal responses to falling plasma glucose concentrations (Figure 2.5) are further illustrated in Figure 2.6. Low plasma glucose concentrations are sensed by

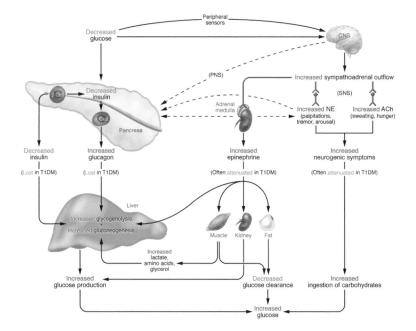

Figure 2.5. Physiological and behavioral defenses against hypoglycemia in humans. ACh, acetylcholine; NE, norepinephrine; PNS, parasympathetic nervous system; SNS, sympathetic nervous system; T1DM, type 1 diabetes. From Cryer 2006b, with permission from the American Society for Clinical Investigation.

pancreatic β-cells, resulting in a decrease in insulin secretion. The resulting decrease in intra-islet insulin, perhaps among other β-cell secretory products, in concert with low glucose levels, signals an increase in α-cell glucagon secretion (Raju and Cryer 2005; Cooperberg and Cryer 2010a; Cryer 2012). Thus, the first and second physiological defenses against falling plasma glucose concentrations—a decrement in insulin secretion and an increment in glucagon secretion—are mediated at the level of the pancreatic islets. Central nervous system (CNS) connections (i.e., innervation) are not required. Because appropriate changes in insulin and glucagon secretion are sufficient to accomplish defense against falling plasma glucose concentrations, the CNS is not normally critical to the prevention or correction of hypoglycemia. However, it becomes critical when the appropriate insulin and glucagon responses do not occur (Chapter 3).

Low plasma glucose concentrations are also sensed in peripheral sites (such as the hepatic portal/mesenteric vein as well as the gut, carotid, body, and oral cavity) and transmitted to the brain and are sensed directly within the brain (Marty et al. 2007; Watts and Donovan 2010). There the hypothalamus initiates an increase in systemic sympathoadrenal activity, including the third physiological defense against falling plasma glucose concentrations—an increment in adrenomedullary epinephrine secretion. That increase in sympathoadrenal activity also includes activation of the sympathetic nervous system and thus, ultimately, the behavioral defense against falling plasma glucose concentrations (the ingestion of carbohydrates). While sympathoadrenal activation tends to decrease insulin secretion and increase glucagon secretion, those insulin and glucagon responses do not require a sympathoadrenal response, since they are also signaled at the level of the pancreatic islets (Raju and Cryer 2005; Cooperberg and Cryer 2010a; Cryer 2012).

There is increasing evidence that the hypothalamic response is modulated by widespread functionally interconnected cerebral inputs (Teves et al. 2004; Arbeláez et al. 2008; Arbeláez et al. 2010), including an inhibitory pathway from the dorsal midline thalamus (Figure 2.6). However, the details of hypothalamic and cerebral mechanisms remain to be determined (Marty et al. 2007; McCrimmon and Sherwin 2010).

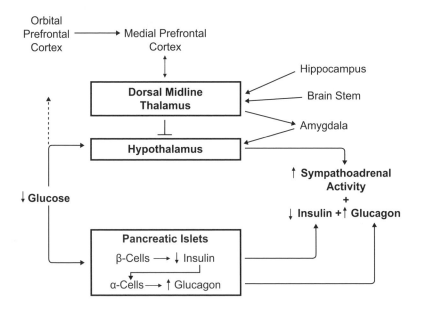

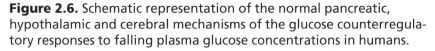

Figure 2.6. Schematic representation of the normal pancreatic, hypothalamic and cerebral mechanisms of the glucose counterregulatory responses to falling plasma glucose concentrations in humans.

At least in part because of the clinical importance of hypoglycemia in people with diabetes, studies of the molecular and cellular physiology and pathophysiology of the CNS-mediated neuroendocrine, including sympathoadrenal, responses to falling plasma glucose concentrations are an increasingly active area of fundamental neuroscience research. Some of these mechanisms have been reviewed (Marty et al. 2007; Cryer 2005; McCrimmon and Sherwin 2010), and these are mentioned in the context of the pathophysiology of glucose counterregulation in diabetes in Chapter 3.

It is interesting that there is only one physiologically effective defense against hyperglycemia, the glucoregulatory hormone insulin, whereas there are redundant physiological and behavioral defenses against hypoglycemia. This may explain why glucoregulatory failure due to relative or absolute insulin deficiency causing hyperglycemia (diabetes mellitus) is common, whereas glucose counterregulatory failure causing hypoglycemia is rare in the absence of drug-treated diabetes. This dichotomy is plausibly explained by evolutionary pressure (Cryer 1997). Typically developing later in life, diabetes would have threatened survival of the individual. In contrast, hypoglycemia would have threatened survival of the species. The irony is that in the setting of demonstrably effective insulin secretagogue or insulin therapy of diabetes, the causative β-cell failure also leads to compromised physiological and behavioral defenses against hypoglycemia (Chapter 3).

Chapter 3.
The Pathophysiology of Glucose Counterregulation in Diabetes

OVERVIEW: INTERPLAY OF INSULIN EXCESS AND COMPROMISED GLUCOSE COUNTERREGULATION

As developed in Chapter 1, iatrogenic hypoglycemia is the limiting factor in the glycemic management of diabetes (Cryer 2004, 2008). It causes recurrent morbidity in most people with type 1 diabetes and many with advanced (absolute endogenous insulin deficient) type 2 diabetes, and is sometimes fatal. In addition, it generally precludes maintenance of euglycemia over a lifetime of diabetes and thus full realization of the vascular benefits of long-term glycemic control. Furthermore, as discussed in this chapter, it compromises defenses against subsequent hypoglycemia and thus causes a vicious cycle of recurrent hypoglycemia.

Hypoglycemia in diabetes is typically the result of the interplay of relative or absolute therapeutic insulin excess and compromised defenses against falling plasma glucose concentrations (Cryer 2004, 2008, 2010, 2011a). Thus, it is fundamentally iatrogenic, the result of treatments that raise circulating insulin levels and thus lower plasma glucose concentrations (Chapter 2). Those treatments include insulin and insulin secretagogues such as a sulfonylurea (e.g., glyburide [glibenclamide], glipizide, glimepiride, or gliclazide, among others) or a glinide (e.g., nateglinide, repaglinide). All people with type 1 diabetes must be treated with insulin. Most people with type 2 diabetes ultimately require treatment with insulin (Turner et al. 1999). Early in the course of the disease, individuals with type 2 diabetes may respond to treatment with an insulin secretagogue. Alternatively, they may respond to drugs that do not raise insulin levels, at least when plasma glucose concentrations fall into and below the physiological range. The latter include a biguanide (metformin), thiazolidinediones (e.g., pioglitazone, rosiglitazone), α-glucosidase inhibitors (e.g., acarbose, miglitol), glucagon-like peptide-1 receptor agonists (e.g., exenatide, liraglutide, lixisenatide), and dipeptidyl peptidase-IV inhibitors (e.g., sitagliptin, saxagliptin, vildagliptin, linagliptin). These drugs should not, and probably do not (Bolen, et al. 2007; Phung et al. 2010; Tschope et al. 2011), cause hypoglycemia when used as monotherapy, although metformin has been reported to cause self-reported hypoglycemia (UKPDS 1995; Wright et al. 2006), or when used in combination among themselves (Chapter 1). However, they can increase the risk of hypoglycemia when used with insulin or with an insulin secretagogue (de Heer and Holst 2007).

INSULIN EXCESS

Relative or even absolute insulin excess must occur from time to time during treatment with an insulin secretagogue or with insulin because of the pharmacokinetic imperfections of these therapies. Even the most sophisticated regimens do not replicate normal (endogenous) insulin secretion, which is plasma glucose regulated and during which variations in circulating insulin levels occur over minutes. With an insulin secretagogue or insulin, to the extent the patient has deficient endogenous insulin secretion, insulin levels are not plasma glucose regulated. Furthermore, variations in insulin levels occur over hours.

Insulin excess of sufficient magnitude can, of course, cause hypoglycemia. However, as developed in Chapter 1, the frequency of hypoglycemia is relatively low (at least with currently recommended glycemic goals) even during therapy with insulin early in the course of type 2 diabetes (UK Hypo Group 2007). (Indeed, it is relatively low very early in the course of type 1 diabetes—the "honeymoon" period.) Therefore, factors in addition to relative or absolute therapeutic insulin excess must play an important role in the pathogenesis of hypoglycemia, which becomes progressively more frequent over time—rapidly in type 1 diabetes and gradually in type 2 diabetes (Chapter 1). Those additional factors are progressive failure of the normal physiological and behavioral defenses against falling plasma glucose concentrations (Chapter 2). Thus, while therapeutic hyperinsulinemia, either relative (to low rates of exogenous or endogenous glucose flux into the circulation or high rates of glucose flux out of the circulation) or absolute, is a prerequisite for the development of hypoglycemia in diabetes, compromised glucose counterregulation is the key feature of the pathogenesis of iatrogenic hypoglycemia in type 1 diabetes and advanced type 2 diabetes. Hypoglycemia in diabetes is typically the result of the interplay of relative or absolute therapeutic insulin excess and compromised physiological and behavioral defenses against falling plasma glucose concentrations (Cryer 2004, 2008, 2010, 2011a).

COMPROMISED GLUCOSE COUNTERREGULATION

As discussed in Chapter 2, the key physiological defenses against falling plasma glucose concentrations (Figure 2.5) are: 1) decrements in pancreatic islet β-cell insulin secretion; 2) increments in pancreatic islet α-cell glucagon secretion, and, absent the latter; 3) increments in adrenomedullary epinephrine secretion (Cryer 2001, 2008, 2010, 2011a). The behavioral defense is the ingestion of carbohydrates prompted by symptoms—largely neurogenic symptoms (DeRosa and Cryer 2004)—that make the individual aware of hypoglycemia (Cryer 2001, 2008, 2010, 2011a). All of these defenses are typically compromised in type 1 diabetes and advanced type 2 diabetes (Cryer 2004, 2008, 2010, 2011a; Dagogo-Jack et al. 1993; Segel et al. 2002).

In fully developed (i.e., C-peptide–negative) type 1 diabetes, circulating insulin levels do not decrease as plasma glucose concentrations decline through or below the physiological range. In the absence of functioning β-cells, plasma insulin levels are simply a passive function of the clearance of administered (exogenous) insulin. Furthermore, in the absence of a β-cell signal, i.e., a decrease in intra-islet insulin perhaps among other β-cell secretory products (Banarer et al. 2002; Raju and Cryer 2005; Gosmanov et al. 2005; Israelian et al. 2005; Cooperberg and Cryer 2009, 2010a; Cryer 2012), circulating glucagon levels do not increase as plasma glucose concentrations fall below the physiological range (Gerich et al. 1973) (Figure 3.1). Thus, both the first defense against hypoglycemia—a decrease in insulin levels—and the second defense against hypoglycemia—an increase in glucagon levels—are lost in type 1 diabetes.

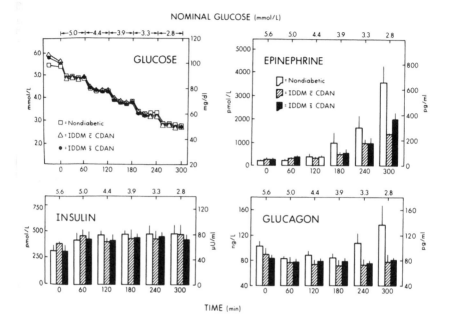

Figure 3.1 Mean (+SE) plasma glucose, insulin, epinephrine, and glucagon concentrations during hyperinsulinemic stepped hypoglycemia glucose clamps in nondiabetic individuals (open squares and columns), people with type 1 diabetes with classical diabetic autonomic neuropathy (CDAN) (open triangles and cross-hatched columns), and people with type 1 diabetes without CDAN (closed circles and columns). From Dagogo-Jack et al. 1993, with permission from the American Society for Clinical Investigation.

Therefore, patients with type 1 diabetes are critically dependent on the third defense against hypoglycemia, an increase in epinephrine levels. However, the epinephrine secretory response to hypoglycemia is typically attenuated in type 1 diabetes (Bolli et al. 1983; Cryer 2004, 2008, 2010, 2011a; Dagogo-Jack et al. 1993) (Figure 3.1). Through mechanisms yet to be clearly defined but often thought to reside in the brain (Cryer 2004, 2005, 2006, 2008, 2010, 2011a), the glycemic threshold for sympathoadrenal—both adrenomedullary and sympathetic neural—activation is shifted to lower plasma glucose concentrations by recent antecedent hypoglycemia (Heller and Cryer 1991b; Dagogo-Jack et al. 1993; Segel et al. 2002) (Figures 3.2 and 3.3), as well as by prior exercise (Galassetti et al. 2001; Sandoval et al. 2004; Ertl and Davis 2004) and by sleep (Jones et al. 1998; Banarer and Cryer 2003; Schultes et al. 2007).

The patterns of plasma insulin, glucagon, and epinephrine responses to falling plasma glucose concentrations in nondiabetic individuals, people with type 1 diabetes, and people with type 2 diabetes are summarized in Table 3.1. The reduced responses to a given level of hypoglycemia cause the clinical syndromes of defective glucose counterregulation and hypoglycemia unawareness (Cryer 2004, 2008, 2010, 2011a).

Defective glucose counterregulation

In the setting of absent decrements in insulin and absent increments in glucagon, attenuated increments in epinephrine as plasma glucose levels fall in response to therapeutic hyperinsulinemia cause the clinical syndrome of defective glucose counterregulation (Cryer 2004, 2008, 2010, 2011a) (Table 3.1). Compared with patients with type 1 diabetes who have absent insulin and glucagon responses but have normal epinephrine responses, patients with absent insulin and glucagon responses and reduced epinephrine responses have been shown to be at 25-fold (White et al. 1983) or greater (Bolli et al. 1984) increased risk for severe iatrogenic hypoglycemia during aggressive glycemic therapy. Originally identified by the failure of glycemic defense against low-dose insulin infusions (White et al. 1983; Bolli et al. 1984), the clinical syndrome of defective glucose counterregulation is characterized by absent decrements in

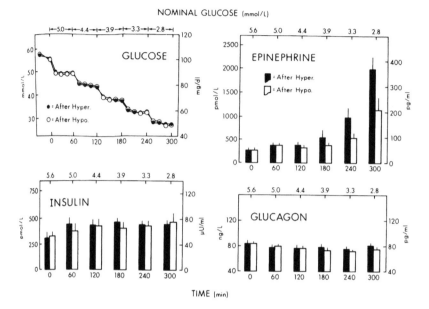

Figure 3.2. Mean (+SE) plasma glucose, insulin, epinephrine, and glucagon concentrations during hyperinsulinemic stepped hypoglycemic glucose clamps in patients with type 1 diabetes (IDDM, insulin dependent diabetes mellitus) without classical diabetic autonomic neuropathy on mornings following afternoon hyperglycemia (After Hyper., closed circles and columns) and on mornings following afternoon hypoglycemia (After Hypo., open circles and columns). From Dagogo-Jack et al. 1993, with permission from the American Society for Clinical Investigation.

insulin, absent increments in glucagon, and attenuated increments in epinephrine at a given level of hypoglycemia in insulin-deficient diabetes (Figure 3.1) (Cryer 2004, 2008, 2010, 2011a; Dagogo-Jack et al. 1993).

Hypoglycemia unawareness

An attenuated epinephrine response to hypoglycemia (Table 3.1) (Figure 3.1) is a marker of an attenuated sympathoadrenal—sympathetic neural as well as adrenomedullary—response.

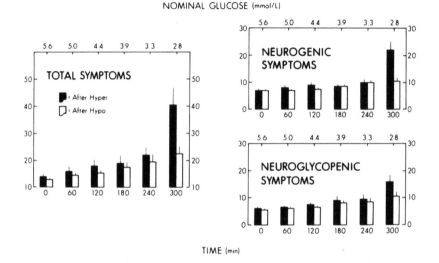

Figure 3.3. Mean (+SE) total, neurogenic, and neuroglycopenic symptom scores during hyperinsulinemic stepped hypoglycemic clamps in patients with type 1 diabetes (IDDM, insulin dependent diabetes mellitus) without classical diabetic autonomic neuropathy on mornings following afternoon hyperglycemia (After hyper., closed columns) and on mornings following afternoon hypoglycemia (After hypo., open columns). From Dagogo-Jack et al. 1993, with permission from the American Society for Clinical Investigation.

Largely as a result of an attenuated sympathetic neural response (DeRosa and Cryer 2004), the attenuated sympathoadrenal response causes the clinical syndrome of hypoglycemia unawareness—impairment or even complete loss of the warning, largely neurogenic symptoms that previously prompted the behavioral defense, the ingestion of carbohydrates. Hypoglycemia unawareness—or more precisely impaired awareness of hypoglycemia—is common in type 1 diabetes, and associated with low plasma glucose concentrations whether those are assessed by A1C levels (Ly et al. 2009) or by continuous glucose

Table 3.1. Responses to Falling Plasma Glucose
Concentrations in Humans

Plasma glucose	Individuals	----------Plasma----------		
—		Insulin	Glucagon	Epinephrine
↓	Non-diabetic	↓	↑	↑
↓	Type 1 diabetes	No ↓	No ↑	Attenuated ↑
		• Defective glucose counterregulation • Hypoglycemia unawareness		
↓	Type 2 diabetes - Early	↓	↑	↑
↓	Type 2 diabetes - Late	No ↓	No ↑	Attenuated ↑

monitoring (Giménez et al. 2009). It is associated with a 6-fold or greater increased risk for severe hypoglycemia (Geddes et al. 2008; Schopman et al. 2010). In one study, patients with type 1 diabetes and impaired awareness of hypoglycemia were found to suffer many more episodes of asymptomatic hypoglycemia than those with intact awareness and were 10-fold more likely (53% vs 5%) to suffer severe hypoglycemia (Schopman et al. 2011). The estimated incidence of severe hypoglycemia was increased from 100 per 100 patient-years in aware individuals to 1600 per 100 patient-years in those with impaired awareness of hypoglycemia.

It is generally thought that hypoglycemia unawareness is due to reduced release of the sympathetic neural neurotransmitters norepinephrine and acetylcholine and perhaps also that of adrenomedullary epinephrine (DeRosa and Cryer 2004).

However, there is evidence of decreased β-adrenergic sensitivity, specifically reduced cardiac chronotropic sensitivity to isoproterenol (Berlin et al. 1987; Fritsche et al. 2001), in patients with unawareness. But vascular sensitivity to infusion of a β2-adrenergic agonist was not found to be reduced in patients with unawareness (de Galan et al. 2006) or following recent antecedent hypoglycemia in nondiabetic individuals (Schouwenberg et al. 2011). Furthermore, reduced symptomatic β-adrenergic sensitivity remains to be demonstrated specifically in patients with unawareness. Finally, it would be necessary also to postulate reduced cholinergic sensitivity to explain reduced cholinergic symptoms such as sweating.

HYPOGLYCEMIA-ASSOCIATED AUTONOMIC FAILURE

Based on the pivotal finding that a 2-hour episode of afternoon hyperinsulinemic hypoglycemia, compared with afternoon hyperinsulinemic euglycemia, reduced the sympathoadrenal and symptomatic (among other) responses to hypoglycemia the following morning in nondiabetic individuals (Heller and Cryer 1991b), the concept of hypoglycemia-associated autonomic failure (HAAF) in diabetes (Cryer 2004, 2008, 2010, 2011a; Dagogo-Jack et al. 1993; Segel et al. 2002; Galassetti et al. 2001; Sandoval et al. 2004; Ertl and Davis 2004; Jones et al. 1998; Banarer and Cryer 2003; Schultes et al. 2007) was formulated (Cryer 1992) and then documented in patients with type 1 diabetes (Dagogo-Jack et al. 1993) and advanced type 2 diabetes (Segel et al. 2002). The effects of prior hypoglycemia on the responses to subsequent hypoglycemia in patients with type 1 diabetes are illustrated in Figures 3.2 and 3.3.

The concept of HAAF in diabetes (Cryer 2004, 2008, 2010, 2011a) posits that recent antecedent hypoglycemia (Dagogo-Jack et al. 1993; Segel et al. 2002; Cryer 2005, 2006b), as well as prior exercise (Galassetti et al. 2001; Sandoval et al. 2004; Ertl and Davis 2004) and sleep (Jones et al. 1998; Banarer and Cryer 2003; Schultes et al. 2007), cause both defective glucose counterregulation (by reducing the adrenomedullary epinephrine response [Figure 3.2] in the absence of decrements in insulin and increments in glucagon) and hypoglycemia unawareness (by reducing the sympathoadrenal, including the sympathetic neural, and the resulting neurogenic symptom responses [Figure 3.3]) and therefore a vicious cycle of recurrent hypoglycemia. The concept of HAAF is illustrated in Figure 3.4.

Absolute therapeutic insulin excess of sufficient magnitude can cause an isolated episode of hypoglycemia even in early T2DM with relative insulin deficiency and therefore, intact insulin and glucagon responses to falling plasma glucose concentrations (Figure 3.4). But, hypoglycemia is infrequent in such individuals. On the other hand, mild to moderate or even relative (to a low rate of glucose influx into the circulation, a high rate of glucose efflux out of the circulation, or both) therapeutic insulin excess often causes hypoglycemia in individuals with absolute endogenous insulin deficiency—advanced type 2 diabetes or type 1 diabetes—and the resulting loss of insulin and glucagon responses to falling plasma glucose levels. In the latter setting, episodes of recent antecedent hypoglycemia, or sleep or prior exercise, result in the addition of an attenuated sympathoadrenal response to falling plasma glucose levels and, thus, the clinical syndromes of defective glucose counterregulation and hypoglycemia unawareness (Figure 3.4) and recurrent iatrogenic hypoglycemia.

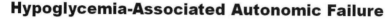

Hypoglycemia-Associated Autonomic Failure

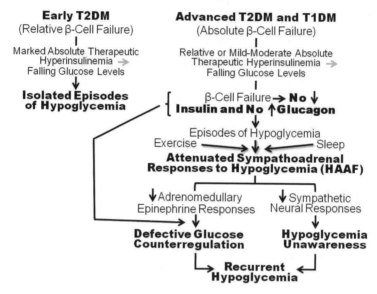

Figure 3.4. Schematic diagram of hypoglycemia-associated autonomic failure (HAAF) in diabetes. Modified from Cryer 2004.

HAAF is a functional disorder distinct from classical diabetic autonomic neuropathy (Dagogo-Jack et al. 1993; Ryder et al. 1990). It is a dynamic phenomenon that can be induced (by prior hypoglycemia or exercise or by sleep) and largely reversed (e.g., by avoidance of hypoglycemia) and is manifested clinically by recurrent iatrogenic hypoglycemia. In contrast, diabetic autonomic neuropathy is a structural disorder that is manifested clinically by gastrointestinal or genitourinary symptoms, by orthostatic hypotension, or by combinations of these and is not reversible. Nonetheless, there is evidence that the key feature of HAAF—an attenuated sympathoadrenal response to a given level of hypoglycemia—is more prominent in patients with diabetic autonomic neuropathy (Bottini et al. 1997; Meyer et al. 1998). That is illustrated in Figure 3.1 (Dagogo-Jack et al. 1993). Indeed, recent antecedent hypoglycemia reduces sympathoadrenal responses to subsequent hemodynamic stimuli, and reduces baroreflex sensitivity (Adler et al. 2009). Thus, HAAF includes a form of autonomic failure functionally analogous to autonomic neuropathy with respect to cardiovascular, as well as metabolic, regulation.

The clinical impact of HAAF is well established in type 1 diabetes (Dagogo-Jack et al. 1993, 1994; White et al. 1983; Bolli et al. 1984; Geddes et al. 2008; Fanelli et al. 1993, 1994b, 1998; Ovalle et al. 1998; Cranston et al. 1994). For example, recent antecedent hypoglycemia, even asymptomatic nocturnal hypoglycemia, reduces epinephrine, symptomatic, and cognitive dysfunction responses to a given level of subsequent hypoglycemia (Fanelli et al. 1998); reduces detection of hypoglycemia in the clinical setting (Ovalle et al. 1998); and reduces glycemic defense against hyperinsulinemia (Dagogo-Jack et al. 1993) in type 1 diabetes. Perhaps the most compelling support for the concept of HAAF is the finding, in three independent laboratories, that as little as 2–3 weeks of scrupulous avoidance of hypoglycemia reverses hypoglycemia unawareness (Figure 3.5) and improves the reduced epinephrine component of defective glucose counterregulation in most affected patients (Fanelli et al. 1993, 1994b; Cranston et al. 1994; Dagogo-Jack et al. 1994). In addition, successful islet transplantation in type 1 diabetes which virtually eliminates a need for therapy with exogenous insulin and thus eliminates iatrogenic hypoglycemia—results in an improved epinephrine response to hypoglycemia, as well as qualitatively appropriate insulin and glucagon responses to hypoglycemia from the graft (Rickels et al. 2011).

Developed initially in type 1 diabetes (Dagogo-Jack et al.

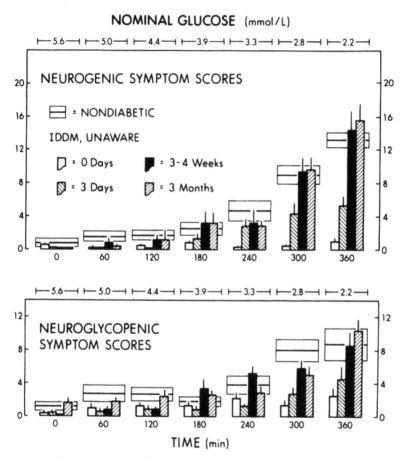

Figure 3.5. Mean (+SE) neurogenic and neuroglycopenic symptom scores during hyperinsulinemic stepped hypoglycemic clamps in non-diabetic individuals (rectangles) and in patients with type 1 diabetes (IDDM, columns) at baseline (0 days), after 3 days of inpatient strict avoidance of hypoglycemia, and after 3–4 weeks and 3 months of outpatient scrupulous avoidance of hypoglycemia. From Dagogo-Jack et al. 1994, with permission from the American Diabetes Association.

1993), the concept of HAAF has been extended to type 2 diabetes (Segel et al. 2002). In advanced (i.e., absolute endogenous insulin deficient) type 2 diabetes, glucagon responses to hypoglycemia are lost (Segel et al. 2002), as they are in type 1 diabetes. Furthermore, the glycemic thresholds for epinephrine and symptom responses (among other responses) are shifted to lower plasma glucose concentrations by recent antecedent hypoglycemia in type 2 diabetes (Segel et al. 2002; Davis et al. 2009), as they are in type 1 diabetes. Thus, people with advanced type 2 diabetes are also at risk for HAAF.

The findings that people with relatively mild type 2 diabetes reasonably but not fully controlled with diet or oral antidiabetic agents have estimated glycemic thresholds for glucose counterregulatory hormone (Spyer et al. 2000; Levy et al. 1998) and symptomatic (Spyer et al. 2000; Choudhary et al. 2009) responses to hypoglycemia at higher plasma glucose concentrations than nondiabetic individuals are likely the result of the pathophysiology of glucose counterregulation in diabetes rather than a unique feature of type 2 diabetes. They are plausibly attributed to the fact that these individuals with type 2 diabetes have higher mean plasma glucose concentrations which raise the glycemic thresholds to higher plasma glucose levels (Amiel et al. 1988; Boyle et al. 1988) (and have fewer episodes of iatrogenic hypoglycemia that would shift the glycemic thresholds to lower plasma glucose levels), as discussed earlier.

In summary, the pathophysiology of glucose counterregulation, and thus the pathogenesis of iatrogenic hypoglycemia, is basically the same in type 1 diabetes and type 2 diabetes. Iatrogenic hypoglycemia is typically the result of the interplay of therapeutic hyperinsulinemia and compromised defenses against falling plasma glucose concentrations (HAAF in diabetes). However, because HAAF stems fundamentally from β-cell failure (Cryer 2008, 2010, 2011a; Raju and Cryer 2005, Cooperberg and Cryer 2010a), which results in loss of both the insulin and glucagon responses, setting the stage for the effect of attenuated sympathoadrenal responses to cause defective glucose counterregulation, as well as hypoglycemia unawareness, it develops rapidly in type 1 diabetes (in which β-cell failure develops rapidly) but slowly in type 2 diabetes (in which absolute β-cell failure develops slowly). That explains the relatively low frequency of hypoglycemia (at least with currently recommended glycemic goals) early in the course of type 2 diabetes and the relatively high frequency of hypoglycemia, approaching that in type 1 diabetes, as patients approach the insulin-deficient end of the spectrum of type 2 diabetes (Chapter 1).

DIVERSE CAUSES OF HAAF

It is now recognized that there are diverse causes of HAAF in diabetes (Cryer 2004, 2008, 2010, 2011a) (Figure 3.4). Those include 1) HAAF induced by recent antecedent iatrogenic hypoglycemia—hypoglycemia-related HAAF (Dagogo-Jack et al. 1993; Segel et al. 2002); 2) HAAF induced by prior exercise—exercise-related HAAF (Galassetti et al. 2001; Sandoval et al. 2004; Ertl and Davis 2004); and 3) HAAF induced by sleep—sleep-related HAAF (Jones et al. 1998; Banarer and Cryer 2003; Schultes et al. 2007). Each of these inciting events causes reduced sympathoadrenal and symptomatic responses to a given level of subsequent hypoglycemia, the key feature of HAAF (i.e., sympathoadrenal failure associated with the development of iatrogenic hypoglycemia in diabetes). Indeed, it is conceivable that there are additional causes of HAAF.

Hypoglycemia-related HAAF

Recent antecedent iatrogenic hypoglycemia was the first recognized cause of HAAF and led to the concept (Cryer 2004, 2008, 2010, 2011a; Dagogo-Jack et al. 1993; Segel et al. 2002) (Figure 3.5). It has been discussed in detail here.

Exercise-related HAAF

Exercise increases glucose utilization (by exercising muscle). In nondiabetic individuals, decrements in insulin, increments in glucagon, and, during intense exercise, increments in catecholamines result in increases in glucose production that generally match, or even exceed, those in glucose utilization, and hypoglycemia does not occur (Ertl and Davis 2004). However, largely because insulin levels are unregulated, hypoglycemia occurs commonly during or shortly after exercise in people with type 1 diabetes (Tansey et al. 2006). Interestingly, the risk of hypoglycemia appears to be higher during late afternoon, compared with prebreakfast, exercise (Ruegemer et al. 1990).

While the risk of hypoglycemia during or shortly after exercise in type 1 diabetes is generally recognized, the risk of late post-exercise hypoglycemia (MacDonald 1987; Tsalikian et al. 2005) is less widely appreciated. Post-exercise late-onset hypoglycemia in type 1 diabetes, typically nocturnal and occurring 6–15 hours after unusually strenuous exercise, was nicely described by MacDonald more than two decades ago (MacDonald 1987). In one more recent study, a quarter of patients with type 1 diabetes suffered nocturnal hypoglycemia in the absence of exercise the previous afternoon and half of the patients suffered nocturnal hypoglycemia after exercise the previous afternoon (Tsalikian et al. 2005). That finding follows directly from the pathophysiology of glucose counterregulation

(Galassetti et al. 2001; Sandoval et al. 2004; Ertl and Davis 2004). Davis and colleagues have reported that exercise reduces sympathoadrenal responses to a given level of hypoglycemia several hours later in both nondiabetic individuals (Galassetti et al. 2001) and people with type 1 diabetes (Sandoval et al. 2004). The latter have absent insulin and glucagon responses and reduced sympathoadrenal and symptomatic responses to hypoglycemia, and their sympathoadrenal responses are reduced further after exercise (Sandoval et al. 2004). They have exercise-related HAAF (Ertl and Davis 2004) and, therefore, an increased risk of hypoglycemia (Tsalikian et al. 2005).

Sleep-related HAAF

In people with type 1 diabetes, sympathoadrenal responses to a given level of hypoglycemia are reduced further during sleep (Jones et al. 1998; Banarer and Cryer 2003). Perhaps because of their further reduced sympathoadrenal responses, they are much less likely to be awakened by hypoglycemia than nondiabetic individuals (Banarer and Cryer 2003; Schultes et al. 2007). Thus, sleeping patients with type 1 diabetes have both further reduced epinephrine responses to hypoglycemia, the key feature of defective glucose counterregulation, and reduced arousal from sleep, a form of hypoglycemia unawareness. They have sleep-related HAAF (Jones et al. 1998; Banarer and Cryer 2003; Schultes et al. 2007) and are at high risk for hypoglycemia (Raju et al. 2006).

Additional causes of HAAF

There may be as yet unrecognized functional, and thus potentially reversible, causes of HAAF in addition to recent antecedent hypoglycemia, prior exercise, and sleep. Furthermore, there may well be a structural factor, since the adrenal medullae can be conceptualized as postganglionic neurons without axons and therefore could be subject to neuropathy (Dagogo-Jack et al. 1993; Bottini et al. 1997; Meyer et al. 1998). Indeed, there are clues to a fixed reduction of the epinephrine response to a given level of hypoglycemia in people with long-standing type 1 diabetes. First, while it reverses hypoglycemia unawareness, scrupulous avoidance of iatrogenic hypoglycemia improves but does not fully normalize the plasma epinephrine response to hypoglycemia (Fanelli et al. 1993, 1994b; Cranston et al. 1994; Dagogo-Jack et al. 1994). Second, when it is successful by producing insulin independence, islet transplantation virtually eliminates hypoglycemia and normalizes the glycemic threshold for epinephrine secretion and increases its magnitude, but it does not appear to fully normalize the magnitude of the epinephrine response (Rickels et al. 2007; Rickels et al. 2011). Third, as mentioned earlier, the epinephrine response to hypoglycemia is reduced to a greater extent in patients with clinically apparent classical diabetic autonomic neuropathy than it is in individuals without overt evidence of that complication (Bottini et al. 1997; Meyer et al. 1998). Fourth, the finding of a reduced plasma metanephrine, as well as epinephrine, response to hypoglycemia in patients with HAAF suggests a reduced adrenomedullary epinephrine secretory capacity (de Galan et al. 2004).

MECHANISMS OF HAAF

HAAF develops in the setting of absent decrements in insulin and absent increments in glucagon as plasma glucose concentrations fall in response to therapeutic hyperinsulinemia in type

1 diabetes and advanced type 2 diabetes (Cryer 2004, 2008, 2010, 2011a). The mechanisms of these prerequisite abnormalities are different from those of the attenuated sympathoadrenal and resulting symptomatic responses to hypoglycemia that ultimately cause the clinical syndromes of defective glucose counterregulation and hypoglycemia unawareness, the components of HAAF, as discussed earlier. These mechanisms are summarized in Figure 3.6.

Absent insulin and glucagon responses

The glucagon rersponse to hypoglycemia is lost in type 1 diabetes (Gerich et al. 1973). It is lost early, before the sympathoadrenal response becomes attenuated (Bolli et al. 1983); indeed, it is lost within the first year of type 1 diabetes (Arbeláez et al. 2012).

Because both type 1 diabetes and advanced (i.e., absolute endogenous insulin deficient) type 2 diabetes are the result of pancreatic islet β-cell failure, the mechanism of the loss of a decrement in insulin as plasma glucose concentrations decline within and below the physiological range is straightforward. That of the loss of the increment in glucagon is less clear-cut (Cryer 2004, 2008, 2010, 2011a, 2012).

Glucagon secretory responses to administered amino acids occur in patients with insulin-deficient diabetes who have no glucagon response to hypoglycemia (Wiethop and Cryer 1993a; Caprio et al. 1993; Hoffman et al. 1994; Rossetti et al. 2008). Therefore, loss of the glucagon response to falling plasma glucose concentrations in type 1 diabetes (Gerich et al. 1973; Bolli et al. 1983; White et al. 1983; Fanelli et al. 1993, 1998; Ovalle et al. 1998; Fukuda et al. 1988; Dagogo-Jack et al. 1993, 1994) and advanced type 2 diabetes (Segel et al. 2002) must be the

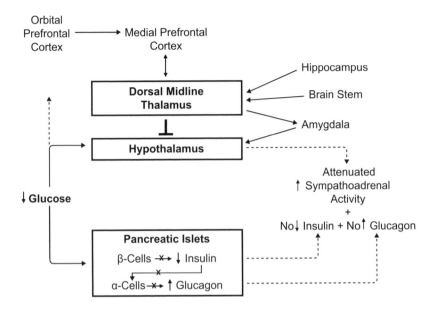

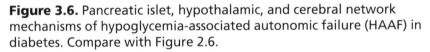

Figure 3.6. Pancreatic islet, hypothalamic, and cerebral network mechanisms of hypoglycemia-associated autonomic failure (HAAF) in diabetes. Compare with Figure 2.6.

result of a defect in signaling to functional glucagon-secreting pancreatic islet α-cells. (The extent to which the reduced absolute glucagon response to administered amino acids in type 1 diabetes [Wiethop and Cryer 1993a; Caprio et al. 1993; Rossetti et al. 2008] is the result of reduced glucagon secretion per α-cell, a reduced α-cell mass, or both is unknown.)

As discussed in Chapter 2, the normal regulation of α-cell glucagon secretion is complex and incompletely understood (e.g., Cooperberg and Cryer 2009, 2010a). However, there is now substantial evidence that β-cell secretory products normally inhibit α-cell glucagon secretion and that a decrease in β-cell secretion, including a decrease in insulin secretion, signals an increase in α-cell glucagon secretion during hypoglycemia in humans (Banarer et al. 2002; Raju and Cryer 2005; Gosmanov et al. 2005; Israelian et al. 2005; Cooperberg and Cryer 2009, 2010a). Thus, it follows that β-cell failure causes loss of the glucagon secretory response to hypoglycemia early in type 1 diabetes and later in type 2 diabetes (Cryer 2004, 2008, 2010, 2011a) (Figure 3.6). That construct is supported by the findings that 1) the degree of loss of glucagon secretion is associated with the degree of loss of insulin secretion (Fukuda et al. 1988); 2) an increase in glucagon secretion can be triggered by a decrease in (exogenous) insulin during hypoglycemia in type 1 diabetes (Cooperberg and Cryer 2010a); and 3) the normal inverse relationship between pulses of insulin and glucagon secretion is lost in type 2 diabetes (Menge et al. 2011).

Loss of the glucagon response to hypoglycemia in absolute endogenous insulin deficient diabetes cannot be attributed to loss of islet nerves (Taborsky et al. 2009) or to loss of CNS-derived neural signaling (McCrimmon and Sherwin 2010). Quantitatively normal glucagon secretory responses to hypoglycemia occur from the denervated (transplanted) human pancreas (Diem et al. 1990) and from the denervated dog pancreas (Sherck et al. 2001) as well as in patients with spinal cord transections and, therefore, no sympathoadrenal outflow to the islets (Palmer et al. 1976). Qualitatively normal glucagon secretory responses to low glucose levels occur from the perfused rodent pancreas (Gerich et al. 1974) and from perifused rodent and human islets (Walker et al. 2011). Furthermore, adrenergic blockade does not prevent the glucagon response to hypoglycemia in humans (Rizza et al. 1979) and epinephrine-deficient bilaterally adrenalectomized individuals have a normal glucagon response to hypoglycemia (DeRosa and Cryer 2004). The role of glucagon in the pathogenesis of hypoglycemia (and hyperglycemia) in diabetes has been reviewed (Cryer 2012).

This intra-islet insulin hypothesis does not include a role for somatostatin, secreted from islet δ-cells, in the physiology or pathophysiology of glucagon secretion. If hypoglycemia decreases somatostatin secretion (Braun et al. 2009), it is conceivable that a decrease in intra-islet somatostatin, as well as insulin, could normally signal increased glucagon secretion and that loss of that signal could explain loss of the glucagon response. Indeed, infusion of a somatostatin antagonist has been reported to increase the glucagon secretory response to hypoglycemia in streptozotocin diabetic rats (Yu et al. 2012). However, selective destruction of β-cells, as in type 1 diabetes, results in both diabetes and loss of the glucagon response to hypoglycemia (Zhou et al. 2007), a finding that seemingly implicates a decrease in intra-islet insulin as the relevant signal to glucagon secretion.

Attenuated sympathoadrenal responses

The mechanism(s) of the key component of HAAF in diabetes, the attenuated central nervous system (CNS)–mediated sympathoadrenal response to falling plasma glucose concentrations, is not known. The attenuated sympathoadrenal response causes hypoglycemia unawareness and, in the setting of absent decrements in insulin and absent increments in glucagon, the attenuated adrenomedullary epinephrine response causes defective glucose counterregulation, and thus HAAF and iatrogenic hypoglycemia in type 1 diabetes and advanced type 2 diabetes (Cryer 2004, 2008, 2010, 2011a; Dagogo-Jack et al. 1993; Segel et al. 2002). Clearly, however, the mechanism is different from that of loss of the insulin and glucagon responses to hypoglycemia, since the latter occur primarily at the level of the diseased pancreatic islets, whereas the attenuated sympathoad-renal response involves the CNS (Figure 3.6).

Theoretically, the alteration that causes the glycemic thresh-olds for the sympathoadrenal and symptomatic (among other) responses to shift to lower plasma glucose concentrations after recent antecedent hypoglycemia (or after exercise and during sleep) could be in the CNS or in the afferent or efferent com-ponents of the sympathoadrenal system. Indeed, the finding of a reduced plasma metanephrine response to hypoglycemia in patients with type 1 diabetes and HAAF suggests a reduced adrenomedullary capacity to secrete epinephrine (de Galan et al. 2004). HAAF is mediated through adrenergic mechanisms (Ramanathan and Cryer 2011). Combined α- and β-adrenergic blockade prevents the effect of hypoglycemia to attenuate the sympathoadrenal response to subsequent hypoglycemia. Inter-estingly, there is evidence that ventromedial hypothalamic β_2-adrenergic stimulation increases the plasma epinephrine response to hypoglycemia in rats (Szepietowska et al. 2011). HAAF may involve decreased glutamate signaling within the hypothalamus (Tong et al. 2007). Potential CNS mechanisms include 1) the systemic mediator hypothesis, 2) the brain fuel transport hypothesis, 3) the brain metabolism hypothesis, and 4) the cerebral network hypothesis (Cryer 2005, 2008, 2010, 2011a; McCrimmon and Sherwin 2010).

The systemic mediator hypothesis posits that increased cir-culating cortisol levels (or perhaps those of another systemic factor) during recent antecedent hypoglycemia (or exercise) act on the brain to reduce the sympathoadrenal (among other) responses to a given level of subsequent hypoglycemia (Davis et al. 1996, 1997a). Substantial antecedent cortisol elevations, produced by cortisol infusion or ACTH administration, do reduce the sympathoadrenal and symptomatic responses to subsequent hypoglycemia (Davis et al. 1996; McGregor et al. 2002). However, that appears to be an effect of supraphysiological cortisol concentrations. Less marked plasma cortisol elevations, to levels comparable to those that occur during hypoglycemia, do not reduce adrenomedullary or symptomatic responses to subsequent hypoglycemia (Raju et al. 2003; Goldberg et al. 2006). Furthermore, inhibition of the cortisol response to antecedent hypoglycemia (with metyrapone) does not prevent the effect of antecedent hypoglycemia to reduce the sympathoadrenal (or other) responses to subsequent hypoglycemia (Goldberg et al. 2006). However, cortisol infusions leading to plasma cortisol concentrations similar to those that occur during hypoglycemia have been reported to blunt sympathoadrenal (among other) responses to subsequent exercise (Bao et al. 2009). There is also evidence that antecedent plasma epinephrine elevations do not cause HAAF (de Galan et al. 2003).

The brain fuel transport hypothesis posits that recent antecedent hypoglycemia causes increased blood-to-brain transport of glucose (or of an alternative metabolic fuel) and thus reduces sympathoadrenal (and other) responses to subsequent hypoglycemia (Cryer 2004, 2008, 2010, 2011a). Early findings were seemingly consistent with the idea of increased blood-to-brain transport of glucose, the primary brain metabolic fuel (Clarke and Sokoloff 1994), in the pathogenesis of HAAF. Hypoglycemia results in increased cerebral vascular expression of GLUT-1 and brain glucose uptake in rodents; however, that requires three days (McCall et al. 1986) or longer (Simpson et al. 1999) of hypoglycemia, much longer than the less than two hours of antecedent hypoglycemia known to reduce the sympathoadrenal response to subsequent hypoglycemia in humans

(Heller and Cryer 1991b). Furthermore, brain glucose uptake, determined with the Kety-Schmidt technique, was reported to be maintained during hypoglycemia with prior hypoglycemia in nondiabetic individuals and in patients with type 1 diabetes with low A1C levels and, thus, likely recent antecedent hypoglycemia; however, in both instances (Boyle et al. 1994, 1995) the difference was greater estimated cerebral blood flows rather than increased glucose arteriovenous differences across the brain. On the other hand, global blood-to-brain glucose transport, measured with [1-^{11}C]glucose positron emission tomography (PET), is not reduced in people with poorly controlled type 1 diabetes (Fanelli et al. 1998) and nearly 24 hours of interprandial hypoglycemia (~55 mg/dl), which reduces the sympathoadrenal and symptomatic responses to subsequent hypoglycemia, does not increase global blood-to-brain glucose transport (or brain glucose metabolism) at the subphysiological plasma glucose concentration of 65 mg/dl (3.6 mmol/l) in healthy individuals (Segel et al. 2001). Furthermore, global blood-to-brain [^{11}C]3-O-methylglucose (Bingham et al. 2005) and [^{18}F]deoxyglucose (Cranston et al. 2001; Dunn et al. 2007) transport, both measured with PET, are not increased in type 1 diabetes patients with hypoglycemia unawareness. In addition, the rate of blood-to-brain glucose transport does not normally determine that of brain glucose metabolism; the former exceeds the latter even at slightly subphysiological plasma glucose concentrations (Fanelli et al. 1998; Segel et al. 2001). As discussed in Chapter 2, the plasma glucose concentration at which glucose transport into the brain becomes limiting to brain glucose metabolism is not known, and may be <54 mg/dl (3.0 mmol/l) (van de Ven et al. 2011). An increase in blood-to-brain glucose transport during hypoglycemia would not be expected to increase brain glucose metabolism, and reduce the glucose counterregulatory response, unless transport were shifted from below to above that glycemic threshold. These findings do not support the notion that increased blood-to-brain glucose transport is the mechanism of HAAF. If it is, the increase would need to be regional. However, the hypothesis was based on global blood-to-brain glucose transport (McCall et al. 1986; Simpson et al. 1999; Boyle et al. 1994, 1995). A variation on this theme would be increased glucose metabolism in the ventromedial hypothalamus in the absence of an increase in blood-to-brain glucose transport (Levin et al. 2008; Kang et al. 2008; Osundiji et al. 2011). Given the finding that prior hypoglycemia did not increase global brain glucose metabolism in humans (Segel et al. 2001), that mechanism would also need to be regional.

The brain can, of course, oxidize alternative fuels. Indeed, neurons normally oxidize lactate as well as glucose but that is largely lactate derived from glucose within the brain—mostly glucose transported from the circulation into the brain but partly that derived from glycogen in astrocytes (Itoh et al. 2003; Hyder et al. 2006). A report of increased blood-to-brain acetate transport in patients with diabetes (Mason et al. 2006)—albeit not in patients with HAAF compared with those without HAAF —raised the possibility that increased transport of a monocarboxylate alternative fuel such as lactate might be involved in the pathogenesis of HAAF. Indeed [3-^{13}C]lactate nuclear magnetic resonance spectroscopy data in rats indicate that hypoglycemia increases brain neural lactate consumption (Herzog et al. 2009) and increased brain lactate concentrations during hypoglycemia have been reported in patients with type 1 diabetes (De Feyter et al. 2012).

The brain metabolism hypothesis posits that recent antecedent hypoglycemia (or sleep or prior exercise) alters the hypothalamic (and hind brain) regulation of the sympathoadrenal response to falling plasma glucose concentrations, resulting in HAAF (Levin et al. 2008; Sherwin 2008; McCrimmon and Sherwin 2010). Interestingly, this basically clinical issue—the mechanism of HAAF—has become a focus of fundamental neuroscience research probing the cellular and molecular mechanisms of the normal brain responses to hypoglycemia and the alterations that might lead to an attenuated sympathoadrenal response following episodes of hypoglycemia. Much of that focus has been on the ventromedial hypothalamus, a key site of the regulation of the sympathoadrenal response to falling glucose levels, and its glucose-excited and glucose-inhibited neurons. Changes that could result in a reduced response include increased glucokinase or KATP channel closure or decreased AMP-activated protein kinase activity and increased GABA or urocortin 3 release (McCrimmon and Sherwin 2010).

A variant of the brain metabolism hypothesis is the notion of brain glycogen supercompensation (Gruetter 2003). If the normally small astrocytic glycogen pool (Chapter 2) increases substantially after hypoglycemia (Choi et al. 2003), that expanded source of glucose (and lactate) within the brain could result in a reduced sympathoadrenal response during subsequent hypoglycemia. However, the evidence in rats that brain glycogen contents increase substantially above baseline after hypoglycemia (Choi et al. 2003) has not been confirmed (Herzog et al. 2008; Canada et al. 2011) and the brain glycogen supercompensation hypothesis has not been supported in humans (Öz et al. 2012). Brain glycogen contents were not increased in patients with type 1 diabetes selected for hypoglycemia unawareness; if anything, they were lower than in controls. Parenthetically, that finding is also inconsistent with the thesis that an increase in blood-to-brain glucose transport causes HAAF. Since brain glycogen synthesis is a direct function of the plasma glucose concentration and blood-to-brain glucose transport, increased blood-to-brain glucose transport should result in increased brain glycogen; that was not the case in patients selected for HAAF.

Three potential pharmacological approaches to reversing HAAF—adrenergic antagonists, a selective serotonin reuptake inhibitor or an opioid receptor antagonist—are of particular interest because they enhance glucose counterregulatory responses to falling plasma glucose concentrations, i.e., the glucose counterregulatory responses become plasma glucose regulated, and they prevent the key feature of HAAF, the attenuated sympathoadrenal response to falling glucose levels (Cryer 2011b). First, combined α-adrenergic and β-adrenergic blockade (demonstrated with the nonselective α and β antagonists phentolamine and propranolol) prevents the effect of hypoglycemia to attenuate the sympathoadrenal response to hypoglycemia the following day in nondiabetic individuals (Ramanathan and Cryer 2011). Second, selective serotonin reuptake inhibitors increase the sympathoadrenal response to hypoglycemia; in diabetic rats sertraline both enhances the plasma epinephrine response to hypoglycemia and prevents the attenuated epinephrine response to subsequent hypoglycemia (Sanders et al. 2008) and in nondiabetic and diabetic humans oral fluoxetine enhances the plasma epinephrine and muscle sympathetic nerve activity responses to hypoglycemia (Briscoe et al. 2008b, 2008a). Third, infusion of the opioid receptor antagonist naloxone increases the plasma epinephrine response to hypoglycemia

(Caprio et al. 1991). When infused during hypoglycemia nalox-one prevents attenuation of the plasma epinephrine, norepi-nephrine, and glucagon responses to hypoglycemia the following day in nondiabetic individuals (Leu et al. 2009) and prevents the further attenuation of the plasma epinephrine response to hypoglycemia the following day in those with type 1 diabetes (Vele et al. 2012a). Furthermore, infusion of nalox-one during exercise has been reported to prevent an attenuated plasma epinephrine response to hypoglycemia the following day in nondiabetic individuals (Milman et al. 2011a). In a subset of subjects with robust plasma β-endorphin responses to exer-cise there was an association between that response and a reduced plasma epinephrine response to hypoglycemia the fol-lowing day in nondiabetic humans (Milman et al. 2012b). Inter-estingly, the magnitude of the plasma β-endorphin response to hypoglycemia was not significantly associated with that of the reduced plasma epinephrine response to hypoglycemia the fol-lowing day in nondiabetic individuals.

Obviously, the brain metabolism and cerebral network hypotheses are not mutually exclusive since alterations in the former may well be components of the latter.

The emerging cerebral network hypothesis posits that recent antecedent hypoglycemia acts through a network of interconnected brain sites to inhibit hypothalamic activation and thus attenuate the sympathoadrenal response, and perhaps contribute to the reduced glucagon response, to subsequent hypoglycemia (Arbeláez et al. 2008). The concept is largely based on findings from neuroimaging of humans during hypo-glycemia, particularly that with [^{15}O]water positron emission tomography ([^{15}O]water PET), which measures regional cere-bral blood flow as an index of regional brain synaptic activity

(Teves et al. 2004; Arbeláez et al. 2008; Teh et al. 2010; Arbeláez et al. 2012), and the psychophysiological concept of habituation of the response to a given recurrent stress and its proposed mechanism. Hypothalamic-pituitary-adrenocortical (HPA) responses to a given stress, such as restraint stress, decrease after repeated exposures to that stress, a phenomenon termed habituation, in rats. The posterior paraventricular nucleus of the thalamus (PVNTh) is a brain site at which previous stress acts to modify responses to subsequent stress in rats (Bhatnagar et al. 2000; Bhatnagar et al. 2002; Jaferi et al. 2003; Grissom and Bhatnagar 2009). Expression of the immediate early gene FosB has been reported to increase in the PVNTh, as well as in hypothalamic sites, during recurrent hypoglycemia in rats (Al-Noori et al. 2008). Based on measurements of plasma epinephrine and norepinephrine concentrations, habituation of the sympathoadrenal system response to repeated restraint stress has also been demonstrated in rats (Konarska et al. 1989; Konarska et al. 1990).

Recent antecedent hypoglycemia has been shown to reduce the sympathoadrenal response to subsequent hypoglycemia in nondiabetic (Heller and Cryer 1991) and diabetic (Dagogo-Jack et al. 1993) humans. That would seem an example of habituation of the sympathoadrenal response in humans. Hypoglycemia has been found to increase synaptic activity in the thalamus, among other brain sites, by three investigative groups (Teves et al. 2004; Arbeláez et al. 2008; Teh et al. 2010; Tesfaye et al. 2011), and to increase synaptic activity to a greater extent during hypoglycemia following recent antecedent hypoglycemia only in the dorsal midline thalamus, the site of the PVNTh (Figure 3.7) (Arbeláez et al. 2008). Indeed, slightly subphysiological plasma glucose concentrations (e.g., 65 mg/dl,

3.5 mmol/l) increase dorsal midline thalamic synaptic activity selectively, or at least predominantly, in humans (Arbeláez et al. 2012). Thus, thalamic activation may be involved in the pathogenesis of the attenuated sympathoadrenal response to hypoglycemia that is the key feature of hypoglycemia-associated autonomic failure (HAAF) in diabetes (Arbeláez et al. 2008).

Inactivation of the medial prefrontal cortex—by microinjection of the GABA-A receptor agonist muscimol—during recurrent restraint has been reported to prevent habituation of the HPA response to that stress in rats (Weinberg et al. 2010). Increased synaptic activity in the medial prefrontal cortex (anterior cingulate) during hypoglycemia has been documented in humans (Teves et al. 2004; Arbelaez et al. 2008; Teh et al. 2010). Thus, the medial prefrontal cortex may also be involved in the cerebral network that results in the attenuated sympathoadrenal response to hypoglycemia that characterizes HAAF in diabetes. Brain sites in addition to the dorsal midline thalamus and the medial prefrontal cortex are undoubtedly involved (Teves et al. 2004; Arbeláez et al. 2008; Teh et al. 2010).

Cranston et al. (2001) found a greater decrease in [^{18}F]deoxyglucose uptake in the subthalamic region of the brain, centered in the hypothalamus, during hypoglycemia in patients with type 1 diabetes and hypoglycemia unawareness. That finding is consistent with the suggestion of increased thalamic inhibition of hypothalamic activity in HAAF (Arbeláez et al. 2008). The description of an array of differences in the patterns of [^{18}F] deoxyglucose uptake during hypoglycemia in patients with type 1 diabetes with and without unawareness (Cranston et al. 2001; Dunn et al. 2007) is consistent with the participation of such a cerebral network in the pathogenesis of HAAF in diabetes.

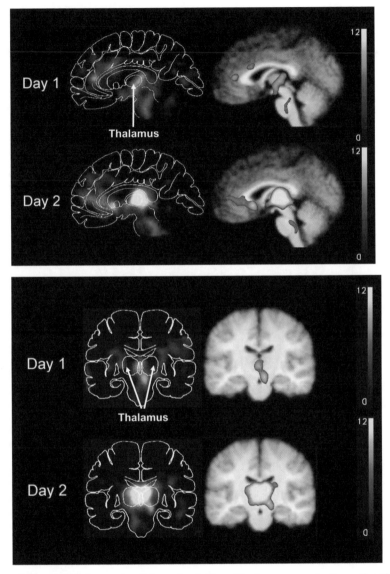

Figure 3.7. Increased dorsal midline thalamus synaptic activation, measured with ¹⁵O water and positron emission tomography, in a model of HAAF in nondiabetic humans. Reproduced from Arbeláez et al. 2008, with permission from the American Diabetes Association.

MECHANISMS OF HYPOGLYCEMIC DEATH: CARDIOVASCULAR HAAF

Although we do not know precisely how often it kills people with diabetes, it is clear that hypoglycemia can kill (Cryer 2011c). First, administration of insulin extract sometimes killed their diabetic dogs, and the Toronto investigators found as early as 1922 that convulsions following insulin administration were associated with low blood glucose concentrations and could be prevented by intravenous glucose administration (Bliss 1982). Furthermore, high mortality rates characterize marked experimental hypoglycemia (Auer 1986; Clarke and Sokoloff 1994; Suh et al. 2007; Reno et al. 2011). Second, hypoglycemia temporally associated with death has been documented in a patient with type 1 diabetes (Tanenberg et al. 2010) (Figure 1.1). In addition, an association between insulin-induced hypoglycemia and cardiac arrhythmias has long been recognized (Goldman 1940) and a patient with hypoglycemia who developed ventricular tachycardia that reverted to sinus rhythm after intravenous glucose administration has been reported (Chelliah 2000). Third, as discussed in Chapter 1, there is an iatrogenic mortality rate in type 1 diabetes. Estimates are that 2 to 10% of patients with type 1 diabetes died from hypoglycemia (Deckert et al. 1978; Tunbridge 1981; Liang et al. 1999; Patterson et al. 2007; DCCT/EDIC 2007; Feltbower et al. 2008; Skrivarhaug et al. 2006). Fourth, hypoglycemic deaths have been reported in many patients with type 2 diabetes (Ferner and Neil 1988; Gerich 1989; Holstein and Egberts 2003). Excess mortality potentially resulting from iatrogenic hypoglycemia has been reported in randomized controlled trials of intensive glycemic therapy in type 2 diabetes (ACCORD 2008) and in hyperglycemic intensive care unit patients (NICE-SUGAR 2009) as well as in type 2 diabetes patients with lower, as well as higher, A1C levels (Currie et al. 2010; Colayco et al. 2011; Huang 2011), as discussed in Chapter 1.

Prolonged, profound hypoglycemia can cause brain death (Auer 1986; Suh et al. 2007a; Cryer 2007; Witsch et al. 2012). Neurons in the cerebral cortex and hippocampus are affected preferentially, followed by those in the basal ganglia and the thalamus in humans. The mechanism of brain death in experimental animals is thought to stem from increased glutamate release and sustained glutamate receptor activation when plasma glucose concentrations are <18 mg/dl (1.0 mmol/l), the EEG is isoelectric, and brain glucose and glycogen levels are unmeasurable. Steps in the pathway from glutamate receptor activation to neuron cell death include Ca2+ influx, mitochondrial calcium deregulation, production of reactive oxygen species, DNA damage, activation of poly(ADP-ribosepolymerase-1 (PARP-1), mitochondrial permeability transition, and mitochondria-to-nucleus translocation of apoptosis-inducing factor (Suh et al. 2007a). PARP-1 inhibitors have been shown to reduce neuronal death (Suh et al. 2003). It has also been reported that high blood glucose concentrations following experimental hypoglycemia can initiate neuronal death by a mechanism involving extracellular zinc release and activation of neuronal NADPH oxidase (Suh et al. 2007b). However, such prolonged, profound hypoglycemia—with plasma glucose concentrations <18 mg/dl (1.0 mmol/l) and an isoelectric EEG— occurs rarely in patients with diabetes. Most fatal hypoglycemic episodes involve other mechanisms, presumably ventricular arrhythmias.

The mechanisms of such fatal hypoglycemic episodes have been reviewed (Lee et al. 2004; Laitinen et al. 2008; Osadchii 2010; Nordin 2010; Frier et al. 2011; Cryer 2011c; Chow and Heller 2012). These could include increased myocardial electrical vulnerability or vascular thromboses. One cardiac mechanism is impaired ventricular repolarization, reflected in a prolonged corrected QT (QTc) interval in the electrocardiogram, which is known to be associated with lethal ventricular arrhythmias. Epinephrine infusion increases the QTc interval (Lee et al. 2003). Insulin-induced hypoglycemia, which causes catecholamine including epinephrine release, increases the QTc interval (Robinson et al. 2003); that effect is blunted by β-adrenergic antagonism with atenolol in nondiabetic persons (Robinson et al. 2003) and patients with type 1 diabetes (Lee et al. 2005). QTc interval prolongation occurs during spontaneous iatrogenic hypoglycemia in people with type 1 diabetes (Gill et al. 2009; Murphy et al. 2004; Robinson et al. 2004) and those with type 2 diabetes (Kalopita et al. 2011). In addition, as a result of the cellular actions of insulin, and of released epinephrine, plasma potassium concentrations decline during insulin-induced hypoglycemia (Caduff et al. 2011). Such QTc interval prolongation and hypokalemia might occur in patients without or with ischemic heart disease or classical diabetic autonomic neuropathy (structural autonomic failure) or those with cardiovascular HAAF (functional autonomic failure). With respect to the latter, compared with hyperinsulinemic euglycemia, hyperinsulinemic hypoglycemia was found to reduce baroreceptor sensitivity, muscle sympathetic nerve activity responses to nitroprusside-induced hypotension, and plasma norepinephrine responses to lower body negative pressure the following day in humans (Adler et al. 2009). That cardiovascular HAAF is entirely analogous to the metabolic HAAF discussed earlier in this chapter.

Given this background, the following concept of the pathogenesis of hypoglycemic mortality (Figure 3.8) (Cryer 2011c) is plausible. Recent antecedent hypoglycemia causes cardiovascular HAAF including reduced baroreflex sensitivity and the resulting increased vulnerability to a ventricular arrhythmia. Recent antecedent hypoglycemia also causes metabolic HAAF with an increased risk for an episode of iatrogenic hypoglycemia with sympathoadrenal activation that could, in the setting of decreased baroreflex sensitivity and through an array of mechanisms including abnormal cardiac repolarization, trigger a ventricular arrhythmia and sudden death. Experimental data support the role of a sympathoadrenal discharge in that combined α- and β-adrenergic blockade reduced deaths of rats during marked hypoglycemia (Reno et al. 2012).

IS HAAF ADAPTIVE OR MALADAPTIVE?

McCrimmon and Sherwin (2010) have expressed the belief that changes in brain metabolism and down regulation of the stress response following recurrent hypoglycemia "are adaptive and not maladaptive and, to that extent this would not be consistent with the current description of this phenomenon as hypoglycemia-associated autonomic failure." Rather, their view is that repeated hypoglycemia induces tolerance of hypoglycemia through preconditioning. That is a plausible view from an evolutionary perspective, and is consistent with 1) the reasoning that it allows individuals to be less troubled by symptoms during hypoglycemia, 2) the evidence of habituation of the hypothalamic-pituitary-adrenocortical response to recurrent restraint

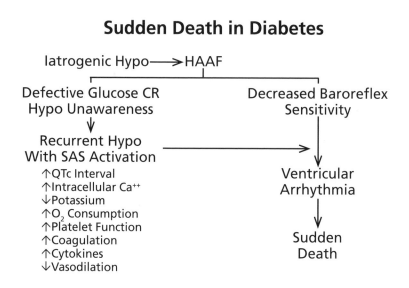

Sudden Death in Diabetes

Figure 3.8. Potential mechanism of iatrogenic hypoglycemia–induced hypoglycemia-associated autonomic failure (HAAF)–mediated sudden death in diabetes: cardiovascular HAAF causing reduced baroreceptor sensitivity and metabolic HAAF causing defective glucose counterregulation (CR) and hypoglycemia (Hypo) unawareness and leading to an episode of hypoglycemia that increases sympathoadrenal system (SAS) activity, which triggers a fatal ventricular arrhythmia in the setting of reduced baroreflex sensitivity. From Cryer 2011c, with permission of the American Journal of Medicine.

stress in rats (Jaferi and Bhatnagar 2006), which could also apply to habituation of the sympathoadrenal response to recurrent hypoglycemic stress in humans (Arbeláez et al. 2008), and 3) the finding that rats subjected to recurrent moderate hypoglycemia had less brain cell death (Puente et al. 2010) and less mortality (Reno et al. 2011) following marked hypoglycemia. However, the concept that recurrent hypoglycemia is adaptive is not plausible from the perspective of a person with diabetes.

Recurrent hypoglycemia causes HAAF in diabetes (Cryer

2006, 2008, 2010, 2011a). HAAF is the sum of defective glucose counterregulation (historically inadequate glucose counterregulation) and hypoglycemia unawareness. Patients with T1DM with defective glucose counterregulation—originally defined as failure to defend the plasma glucose concentration during low-dose insulin infusion (~0.7 mU • kg⁻¹ • min⁻¹) and associated with attenuated plasma epinephrine responses to hypoglycemia—are at 25-fold (White et al. 1983) or even greater (Bolli et al. 1984) increased risk of severe iatrogenic hypoglycemia compared with those with normal glycemic defense against such hyperinsulinemia and normal epinephrine responses. Furthermore, defective glucose counterregulation—again, defined as failure to defend plasma glucose during low dose insulin infusion—and attenuated epinephrine responses to hypoglycemia characterize patients with a history of severe iatrogenic hypoglycemia (Sjöbom et al. 1989). In addition, patients with type 1 diabetes and impaired awareness of hypoglycemia are at about 6-fold increased risk of severe hypoglycemia (Geddes et al. 2008). Those with insulin-treated type 2 diabetes and impaired awareness of hypoglycemia have been reported to be at 17-fold increased risk of severe iatrogenic hypoglycemia (Schopman et al. 2010). Thus, HAAF is clearly maladaptive from the perspective of people with absolute endogenous insulin deficiency, those with type 1 diabetes and advanced type 2 diabetes. In such individuals HAAF increases the risk of severe iatrogenic hypoglycemia, with its morbidity and potential mortality, substantially (White et al. 1983; Bolli et al. 1984; Sjöbom et al. 1989; Geddes et al. 2008; Schopman et al. 2010).

Nonetheless, the findings of Puente et al. (2010) and Reno et al. (2011) indicate that recurrent hypoglycemia reduces seizures, necrosis of brain neurons, cognitive dysfunction, and death following marked hypoglycemia in rats. Thus, it may be that recurrent iatrogenic hypoglycemia is both adaptive, in that it renders patients less vulnerable to the devastating effects of subsequent episodes of hypoglycemia, and maladaptive, in that it renders patients more prone to subsequent hypoglycemia with its morbidity and potential mortality (Reno et al. 2011). The reduced intensity of the typical sympathoadrenal response to hypoglycemia after prior hypoglycemia (Heller and Cryer 1991b; Dagogo-Jack et al. 1993) might be relevant to that reduced vulnerability. However, that does not preclude a massive and potentially fatal ventricular arrhythmia generating sympathoadrenal response to a given episode of very marked hypoglycemia.

SUMMARY

Insulin excess of sufficient magnitude can cause iatrogenic hypoglycemia. However, in the vast majority of instances, it is the integrity of physiological and behavioral defenses against falling plasma glucose concentrations that determines whether an episode of relative, or even absolute, therapeutic hyperinsulinemia results in an episode of hypoglycemia. Thus, hypoglycemia is typically the result of the interplay of therapeutic insulin excess and compromised glycemic defenses (i.e., HAAF) in type 1 diabetes and advanced type 2 diabetes. The common denominator of the two components of HAAF—defective glucose counterregulation and hypoglycemia unawareness—is an attenuated sympathoadrenal response to a given level of hypoglycemia. In addition to therapeutic hyperinsulinemia, absent decrements in insulin and absent increments in glucagon, both the result of β-cell failure in type 1 diabetes and advanced type

2 diabetes, are prerequisites for defective glucose counterregulation. In that setting, attenuated epinephrine responses cause that clinical syndrome. Attenuated sympathoadrenal responses, largely reduced sympathetic neural responses, also cause the clinical syndrome of hypoglycemia unawareness. The attenuated sympathoadrenal responses, the key feature of HAAF, can be caused by recent antecedent hypoglycemia, prior exercise, or sleep, perhaps among other causes. The fact that loss of the insulin and glucagon responses stems from β-cell failure explains why HAAF develops early in the course of type 1 diabetes but only later in the course of type 2 diabetes. That in turn explains why iatrogenic hypoglycemia becomes limiting to glycemic control early in type 1 diabetes but later in type 2 diabetes. Decreased baroreflex sensitivity, a feature of cardiovascular HAAF, may set the stage for a fatal ventricular arrhythmia triggered by the sympathoadrenal response to a subsequent episode of hypoglycemia, the result of metabolic HAAF. Finally, it is conceivable that HAAF both makes patients with diabetes more prone to recurrent hypoglycemia and less vulnerable to the devastating effects of hypoglycemia.

Understanding of this pathophysiology of glucose counterregulation in diabetes leads directly to insight into the risk factors for (Chapter 4), the definition and classification of (Chapter 5), and the prevention or treatment of (Chapter 6) clinical iatrogenic hypoglycemia in diabetes.

Chapter 4.
The Risk Factors for Hypoglycemia in Diabetes

The risk factors for hypoglycemia in people with diabetes (Cryer et al. 2003; Cryer 2004, 2008, 2010, 2011a) (Table 4.1) follow directly from the pathophysiology of glucose counterregulation in diabetes (Chapter 3). The principle is that iatrogenic hypoglycemia in type 1 diabetes and advanced type 2 diabetes is typically the result of the interplay of relative or absolute therapeutic insulin excess and compromised physiological and behavioral defenses against falling plasma glucose concentrations, i.e., hypoglycemia-associated autonomic failure (HAAF) in diabetes.

People with diabetes are not immune to hypoglycemia caused by mechanisms other than the treatment of their diabetes (Cryer et al. 2009). Those include 1) an array of drugs (Murad et al. 2009; Ben Salem et al. 2011) including alcohol, 2) critical illnesses such as renal, hepatic or cardiac failure, sepsis, or inanition, 3) hormone deficiency states such as adrenocortical failure, 4) nonislet tumor hypoglycemia, 5) endogenous hyperinsulinism, and 6) accidental, surreptitious, or even malicious hypoglycemia. However, aside from drug effects, those mechanisms are very uncommon.

RELATIVE OR ABSOLUTE INSULIN EXCESS

The conventional risk factors for hypoglycemia in diabetes (Cryer et al. 2003; Cryer 2004, 2008, 2010, 2011a) are based on the premise that relative or absolute therapeutic insulin excess is the sole determinant of risk. That may be either endogenous (sulfonylurea, or glinide, stimulated) or exogenous insulin excess. People with type 2 diabetes using a sulfonylurea or a glinide and people with type 1 diabetes or type 2 diabetes using

Table 4.1. Risk Factors for Hypoglycemia in Diabetes

Relative or absolute insulin excess:

1. Insulin or insulin secretagogue doses are excessive, ill-timed, or of the wrong type.

2. Exogenous glucose delivery is decreased (e.g., after missed meals and during the overnight fast).

3. Endogenous glucose production is decreased (e.g., after alcohol ingestion).

4. Glucose utilization is increased (e.g., during and shortly after exercise).

5. Sensitivity to insulin is increased (e.g., after weight loss or improved glycemic control and in the middle of the night).

6. Insulin clearance is decreased (e.g., with renal failure).

Hypoglycemia-associated autonomic failure (defective glucose counterregulation and hypoglycemia unawareness):

1. Absolute endogenous insulin deficiency

2. A history of severe hypoglycemia, hypoglycemia unawareness, or both as well as recent antecedent hypoglycemia, prior exercise, and sleep

3. Aggressive glycemic therapy per se (lower A1C levels, lower glycemic goals, or both)

insulin are at ongoing risk for episodes of hyperinsulinemia because of the pharmacokinetic imperfections of those therapies. Indeed, therapeutic hyperinsulinemia is a prerequisite for the development of hypoglycemia in diabetes (Chapter 3). Whereas those episodes can include absolute hyperinsulinemia, the conventional risk factors also focus on relative hyperinsulinemia, i.e., insulin levels insufficient to cause hypoglycemia under most conditions but high enough to cause hypoglycemia in the setting of decreased exogenous glucose delivery or endogenous glucose production, increased glucose utilization, or increased sensitivity to insulin (Table 4.1).

Absolute or relative therapeutic insulin excess occurs when sulfonylurea, glinide, or insulin doses are excessive, ill-timed, or of the wrong type. Relative insulin excess occurs under a variety of conditions. It occurs when exogenous glucose delivery is decreased, as it is after missed (or low-carbohydrate) meals and during the overnight fast; when endogenous glucose production is decreased, as it is after alcohol ingestion; when glucose utilization is increased, as it is during or shortly after exercise; and when sensitivity to insulin is increased, in the long term after weight loss or improved glycemic control and in the short term in the middle of the night. Insulin clearance is decreased with renal failure. Alcohol causes hypoglycemia by inhibiting gluconeogenesis (Cryer et al. 2009). Consumption of alcohol in the evening has been shown to cause hypoglycemia the following morning in patients with type 1 diabetes (Turner et al. 2001).

These are the risk factors people with diabetes and their caregivers deal with whenever hypoglycemia becomes a problem. Clearly, in a given patient, each of these needs to be considered carefully and the regimen adjusted appropriately.

Nonetheless, aside from the first, these risk factors explain only a minority of episodes of hypoglycemia (DCCT 1991). In most instances, other risk factors, specifically those indicative of HAAF, determine whether a given episode of therapeutic hyperinsulinemia does, or does not, result in an episode of hypoglycemia (Chapter 3).

HYPOGLYCEMIA-ASSOCIATED AUTONOMIC FAILURE

The risk factors for hypoglycemia indicative of HAAF (Cryer et al. 2003; Cryer 2004, 2008, 2010, 2011a) (Table 4.1) include the degree of absolute endogenous insulin deficiency (Fukuda et al. 1998; DCCT 1997; Mühlhauser et al. 1998; Allen et al. 2001; Steffes et al. 2003; UK Hypo Group 2007); a history of severe hypoglycemia, hypoglycemia unawareness, or both (DCCT 1997; Mühlhauser et al. 1998; Allen et al. 2001; Wright et al. 2006) and conditions known to cause HAAF (recent antecedent hypoglycemia, prior exercise, or sleep); and aggressive glycemic therapy per se (DCCT 1997; Mühlhauser et al. 1998; Allen et al. 2001; Steffes et al. 2003; Wright et al. 2006; Lüddeke et al. 2007; Hemmingsen et al. 2011).

As discussed earlier, defective glucose counterregulation, one of the components of HAAF, develops in the setting of absent decrements in insulin and absent increments in glucagon, and both of these pathophysiological features stem fundamentally from β-cell failure (Chapter 3). Thus, the degree of absolute endogenous insulin deficiency determines both the extent to which insulin levels will not decrease and the extent to which glucagon levels will not increase as plasma glucose concentrations fall in response to therapeutic hyperinsulinemia.

Longer duration of diabetes is associated with loss of endogenous insulin secretion, early in type 1 diabetes and later in type 2 diabetes. The extent to which age per se (as compared to duration of diabetes and progressive deterioration of β-cell function) plays a role is unclear, but rather subtle abnormalities of glucose counterregulatory defenses have been reported in older people (Marker et al. 1992; Meneilly et al. 1994).

A history of severe hypoglycemia indicates, and a history of hypoglycemia unawareness implies, recent antecedent hypoglycemia. As discussed earlier (Chapter 3), recent antecedent hypoglycemia causes an attenuated sympathoadrenal response to subsequent hypoglycemia, the key feature of defective glucose counterregulation and the cause of hypoglycemia unawareness, which are the two components of HAAF, and thus the pathogenesis of iatrogenic hypoglycemia. In addition to recent antecedent hypoglycemia, prior exercise and sleep cause HAAF.

As documented in clinical trials with sample sizes large enough to demonstrate beneficial effects in type 1 diabetes (DCCT 1993; Reichard and Pihl 1994) and type 2 diabetes (Wright et al. 2006; ADVANCE 2008; ACCORD 2008; Duckworth et al. 2009), and confirmed in a meta-analysis that included 12 smaller trials in type 1 diabetes (Egger et al. 1997), if all other factors are the same, patients treated to lower, compared with higher, A1C levels are at higher risk for hypoglycemia. Stated differently, studies with a control group treated to a higher A1C level consistently report higher rates of hypoglycemia in the group treated to a lower A1C level in type 1 diabetes (DCCT 1993; Reichard and Pihl 1994; Egger et al. 1997) and type 2 diabetes (Wright et al. 2006; ADVANCE 2008; ACCORD 2008; Duckworth et al. 2009). Indeed, lower mean plasma glucose concentrations and greater plasma glucose variability are also associated with a higher risk of hypoglycemia (Kilpatrick et al. 2007). That does not, of course, mean that one cannot both improve glycemic control and minimize the risk for hypoglycemia in individual patients (Cryer et al. 2003; Cryer 2004, 2008, 2010, 2011a; Rossetti et al. 2008) (Chapter 6).

These risk factors for HAAF also apply to young children with T1DM (Brambilla et al. 1987; Jones et al. 1991).

Improved glycemic control before and during pregnancy is particularly important in the short term because it improves pregnancy outcomes in women with type 1 diabetes. But, it increases the frequency of hypoglycemia substantially (Evers et al. 2002; Nielsen et al. 2008; Robertson et al. 2009; Heller et al. 2010). In one series, 45% of 108 women with type 1 diabetes suffered severe hypoglycemia during their pregnancies; compared with a prepregnancy rate of 110 per 100 patient-years, the incidence was the equivalent of 530, 240, and 50 episodes per 100 patient-years in the first, second, and third trimesters, respectively (Neilsen et al. 2008). The risk factors for HAAF—previous severe hypoglycemia (Evers et al. 2002; Nielsen et al. 2008), impaired awareness of hypoglycemia (Nielsen et al. 2008), and lower A1C levels (Evers et al. 2002)—are also associated with higher rates of severe hypoglycemia in pregnant women with type 1 diabetes.

A relationship between the deletion (D) allele of the angiotensin converting enzyme (ACE) gene and its associated higher serum ACE activity and severe hypoglycemia has been reported in some (Pedersen-Bjergaard et al. 2001; Nordfeldt and Samuelson 2003; Pedersen-Bjergaard et al. 2009), but not all (Bulsara et al. 2007; Johannesen et al. 2011) studies in type 1 diabetes. It has also been reported in some (Davis et al. 2011) but not all (Freathy et al. 2006) studies in type 2 diabetes with a weak relationship in another study in type 2 diabetes (Zammitt et al. 2007). The mechanism of this apparent association is unclear. It has been noted that healthy individuals (Pedersen-Bjergaard et al. 2008) and patients with type 1 diabetes (Høi-Hansen et al. 2009) with higher serum ACE activities are more susceptible to cognitive dysfunction during hypoglycemia, a plausible factor in the pathogenesis of severe hypoglycemia. In one contrast of nine patients with T1DM and high renin-angiotensin system (RAS) activity and nine patients with low RAS activity, the high RAS group had reduced symptoms of hypoglycemia, had a 10-fold higher incidence of prior severe hypoglycemia, and tended to have lower glucagon and epinephrine responses to hypoglycemia (Høi-Hansen et al. 2009). Thus, it is conceivable that conventional mechanisms (i.e., HAAF) explain the high frequency of severe hypoglycemia and that the higher serum ACE activity might be a result rather than the cause of hypoglycemia. However, that would not explain the association of severe hypoglycemia with the DD genotype observed in some studies (Pedersen-Bjergaard et al. 2001; Davis et al. 2011).

Chapter 5.
The Clinical Definition and Classification of Hypoglycemia in Diabetes

THE GLUCOSE ALERT VALUE

The American Diabetes Association (ADA) Workgroup on Hypoglycemia (2005) defined hypoglycemia in diabetes as "all episodes of abnormally low plasma glucose concentration that expose the individual to potential harm." That includes asymptomatic hypoglycemia because that also impairs defense against subsequent hypoglycemia (Heller and Cryer 1991b; Fanelli et al. 1998; Davis et al. 1997b). Because the glycemic threshold for symptoms, among other responses to hypoglycemia, shift to lower plasma glucose concentrations in patients with recurrent hypoglycemia and to higher plasma glucose concentrations in those with poorly controlled diabetes (Amiel et al. 1988; Boyle et al. 1988; Mitrakou et al. 1993), it is not possible to state a single plasma glucose concentration that defines hypoglycemia. Nonetheless, the ADA workgroup recommended that people with drug-treated diabetes (implicitly those treated with a sulfonylurea, a glinide, or insulin) become concerned about developing hypoglycemia at a self-monitored plasma glucose concentration of ≤70 mg/dl (≤3.9 mmol/l) (ADA Workgroup on Hypoglycemia 2005). Within the error of self–plasma glucose monitoring (or continuous glucose monitoring) devices, that glucose level approximates the lower limit of the nondiabetic postabsorptive plasma glucose concentration range (Cryer

2001) and the normal glycemic thresholds for activation of physiological glucose counterregulatory systems (Cryer 2001) (Chapter 2), and is low enough to reduce glycemic defenses against subsequent hypoglycemia (Davis et al. 1997b), in nondiabetic individuals. That glucose level is higher than the plasma glucose levels required to produce neurogenic and neuroglycopenic symptoms (50–55 mg/dl, 2.8–3.0 mmol/l) or to impair brain function in nondiabetic individuals (Cryer 2001, 2007) and substantially higher than the glucose levels that do so in people with well-controlled diabetes (Cryer 2007; Amiel et al. 1988), although people with poorly controlled diabetes sometimes have symptoms at somewhat higher glucose levels (Amiel et al. 1988; Boyle et al. 1988).

Use of a 70 mg/dl (3.9 mmol/l) plasma glucose alert level generally gives the patient time to take action to prevent a clinical hypoglycemic episode. Also, in practice, self–plasma glucose monitoring is usually done with devices that are not precise analytical instruments, particularly at low glucose levels (Diabetes Research in Children Network Study Group 2003). The recommended alert level provides some margin for their inaccuracy.

The recommended generic alert level does not mean that people with diabetes should always self-treat at an estimated plasma glucose concentration of ≤70 mg/dl. Rather, it indicates that they should consider actions ranging from repeating the measurement in the short term through behavioral changes, such as avoiding exercise or driving, to carbohydrate ingestion and subsequent regimen adjustments.

The plasma glucose alert value of ≤70 mg/dl (≤3.9 mmol/l) has been criticized as being too high because glucose levels are occasionally lower than that in nondiabetic individuals and its use would lead to an overestimation of the frequency of clinically important hypoglycemia (Amiel et al. 2008). The former is true, especially in women and children. The latter criticism is wide of the mark. The issue is not to estimate the frequency of clinically important hypoglycemia. It is to prevent clinically important hypoglycemia. Notably, after criticizing the ADA recommended alert value, Amiel and colleagues recommended a lower limit of the therapeutic plasma glucose concentration of 72–81 mg/dl (4.0–4.5 mmol/l). Thus, there is really rather little disagreement on this ostensibly contentious issue (Cryer 2009).

CLASSIFICATION OF HYPOGLYCEMIA

The ADA Workgroup also recommended a classification of hypoglycemia in diabetes (ADA Workgroup on Hypoglycemia 2005) (Table 5.1). That includes severe hypoglycemia, using a definition that has been used widely since the initial report of the Diabetes Control and Complications Trial (DCCT 1993), documented symptomatic hypoglycemia, and asymptomatic hypoglycemia, as well as probable symptomatic hypoglycemia and relative hypoglycemia. The latter category reflects the fact that patients with poorly controlled diabetes can experience symptoms of hypoglycemia as their plasma glucose concentrations fall into the physiological range (Amiel et al. 1988; Boyle et al. 1988).

QUANTITATION OF HYPOGLYCEMIA UNAWARENESS

Hypoglycemia unawareness, or impaired awareness of hypoglycemia (IAH) since there is a spectrum from normal awareness through reduced awareness to complete unawareness (Frier and Fisher 1999), is a component of HAAF (Chapter 3) and a risk factor for iatrogenic hypoglycemia (Chapter 4). Three methods have been used to attempt to systematically identify affected patients. The method of Gold et al. (1994) asks the patient to complete a seven-point scale ranging from 1, always aware, to 7, never aware, in response to the question, "Do you know when your hypos are commencing?" A score of ≥4 is considered to indicate impaired awareness of hypoglyce-

Table 5.1. American Diabetes Association Workgroup on Hypoglycemia Classification of Hypoglycemia in People with Diabetes

---

Severe hypoglycemia. An event requiring assistance of another person to actively administer carbohydrate, glucagon, or other resuscitative actions. Plasma glucose measurements may not be available during such an event, but neurological recovery attributable to the restoration of plasma glucose to normal is considered sufficient evidence that the event was induced by a low plasma glucose concentration.

Documented symptomatic hypoglycemia. An event during which typical symptoms of hypoglycemia are accompanied by a measured plasma glucose concentration ≤70 mg/dl (≤3.9 mmol/l).

Asymptomatic hypoglycemia. An event not accompanied by typical symptoms of hypoglycemia but with a measured plasma glucose concentration ≤70 mg/dl (≤3.9 mmol/l).

Probable symptomatic hypoglycemia. An event during which symptoms typical of hypoglycemia are not accompanied by a plasma glucose determination but that was presumably caused by a plasma glucose concentration ≤70 mg/dl (≤3.9 mmol/l).

Relative hypoglycemia. An event during which the person with diabetes reports any of the typical symptoms of hypoglycemia and interprets those as indicative of hypoglycemia, with a measured plasma glucose concentration >70 mg/dl (>3.9 mmol/l) but approaching that level.

mia. The method of Clarke et al. (1995) asks eight questions about the patient's hypoglycemia experience. A score of ≥4 is considered to indicate impaired awareness of hypoglycemia. A score of ≤2 is considered to indicate awareness of hypoglycemia, leaving a score of 3 as not classifiable. The method of Pedersen-Bjergaard (2003) asks the patient to select one of the terms "always," "usually," "occasionally," or "never" in response to the question, "Do you recognize symptoms, when you have a hypo?" Subjects who answer "always" are classified as having normal awareness, those answering "usually" as having impaired awareness, and those answering "occasionally" or "never" as being unaware. Thus, the method of Gold classifies patients as being aware or having impaired awareness, that of Clarke also classifies patients as being aware or having impaired awareness but leaves some patients not classified, and the method of Pedersen-Bjergaard classifies patients as being aware, having impaired awareness, or being unaware (Table 5.2).

An analysis of the application of all three methods to 372

Table 5.2. Proportion of 372 patients with type 1 diabetes classified as having intact awareness of hypoglycemia (Aware), impaired awareness of hypoglycemia (Impaired Awareness), or hypoglycemia unawareness (Unaware) using three methods (Høi-Hansen et al. 2010).

Method	Aware	Impaired Awareness	Unaware
A. Gold, 1994	75%	25%	—
B. Clarke, 1995	51%	28% (21% Not Classified)	—
C. Pedersen-Bjergaard, 2003	41%	46%	13%

patients within type 1 diabetes (Høi-Hansen et al. 2010) is shown in Table 5.2. Patients with impaired awareness or unawareness by all three methods reported 1) fewer neurogenic, but not neuroglycopenic, symptoms of hypoglycemia, 2) symptoms at lower self-monitored plasma glucose concentrations, and 3) higher rates of severe iatrogenic hypoglycemia. Compared with those with awareness, patients classified as having impaired awareness of hypoglycemia by the methods of Gold, Clarke, and Pedersen-Bjergaard reported 3-fold, 6-fold and 8-fold higher rates of severe hypoglycemia, respectively. Those classified as unaware by the method of Pederson-Bjergaard reported a 21-fold higher rate of severe hypoglycemia. Thus, all three methods identify patients at increased risk of severe iatrogenic hypoglycemia. The methods of Gold and of Petersen-Bjergaard offer simplicity. Because impaired awareness/ unawareness is an inducible and reversible phenomenon (Chapter 3), none of the rather diverse proportions shown in Table 5.2 should be taken too literally.

QUANTITATION OF ENDOGENOUS INSULIN DEFICIENCY

Normally, insulin secretion adapts to maintain plasma glucose concentrations within, or return them to, the postabsorptive physiological range. Insulin is secreted from pancreatic β-cells into the hepatic portal venous circulation, and ~50% is cleared by the liver. C-peptide, the peptide cleaved from proinsulin to yield insulin, is secreted in equimolar quantities with insulin. But C-peptide is not cleared by the liver. Therefore, plasma C-peptide concentrations provide an index of endogenous insulin secretion. Indeed, plasma C-peptide data can be used to calculate rates of insulin secretion (Eaton et al. 1980; Polonsky et al. 1986; Heller and Cryer 1991a).

Plasma C-peptide concentrations are ~0.5–1.5 ng/ml (~0.2–0.5 nmol/l) after an overnight fast in healthy euglycemic individuals. Normally, the concentrations decrease as plasma glucose levels decline within the physiological range and become virtually indistinguishable from zero if glucose levels fall below the physiological range (Heller and Cryer 1991a).

One approach to the quantitation of endogenous insulin deficiency is to define the plasma C-peptide concentrations that identify patients with clinical type 1 diabetes. In general, fasting plasma C-peptide concentrations ≤0.6 ng/ml (≤0.2 nmol/l) characterize type 1 diabetes (DCCT 1986; Gjessing et al. 1989; Service et al. 1997), although a higher cutoff value has been reported (Berger et al. 2000) (Table 5.3). A wider range of glucagon-stimulated plasma C-peptide levels has been reported to identify type 1 diabetes (DCCT 1986; Gjessing et al. 1989; Service et al. 1997; Berger et al. 2000) (Table 5.3).

Interestingly, among the 262 patients judged clinically to have type 2 diabetes by Service and colleagues (Service et al. 1997), 20 (8%) displayed an insulin-deficient plasma C-peptide pattern initially, and an additional 33 (13%) did so on at least one occasion during subsequent testing. Unfortunately, the proportion of those patients who had late-onset autoimmune diabetes (i.e., type 1 diabetes), as opposed to progression of type 2 diabetes to absolute endogenous insulin deficiency, is not known.

Absolute insulin deficiency and the resulting absence of a decrease in insulin secretion (and of an increase in glucagon secretion) is a fundamental feature of defective glucose counterregulation and thus HAAF (Chapter 3) and is a risk factor for

Table 5.3. Fasting, Stimulated (6 Minutes after 1.0 mg of Glucagon Intravenously), and Random Plasma C-peptide Concentrations in Patients Judged Clinically to Have Type 1 Diabetes

	Fasting	Stimulated	Random
DCCT 1986	≤0.6 ng/ml	≤1.5 ng/ml	—
	≤0.2 nmol/l	≤0.5 nmol/l	—
Gjessing et al. 1989	<0.6 ng/ml	<1.0 ng/ml	—
	<0.2 nmol/l	<0.3 nmol/l	—
Service et al. 1997	<0.5 ng/ml	↑<0.2 ng/ml	—
	<0.2 nmol/l	↑<0.1 nmol/l	—
Berger et al. 2000	≤1.2 ng/ml	≤1.8 ng/ml	≤1.5 ng/ml
	≤0.4 nmol/l	≤0.6 nmol/l	≤0.5 nmol/l

iatrogenic hypoglycemia (Chapter 4). A subset of patients with type 1 diabetes retain some, albeit still subnormal, insulin secretion. That is relevant to defense against falling plasma glucose concentrations. For example, the proportion of patients who suffered severe hypoglycemia in the DCCT was about 50% lower in the 11% of the patients who had plasma C-peptide concentrations >0.6 ng/ml) (0.2 nmol/l) during a mixed meal at baseline and at least one year later (Steffes et al. 2003).

Chapter 6.
The Prevention and Treatment of Hypoglycemia in Diabetes

PREVENTION OF HYPOGLYCEMIA: HYPOGLYCEMIA RISK FACTOR REDUCTION

It is, of course, preferable to prevent, rather than to treat, hypoglycemia in people with diabetes. The prevention of hypoglycemia requires the practice of hypoglycemia risk factor reduction (Cryer et al. 2003; Cryer 2008). That involves four steps: 1) Acknowledge the problem. 2) Apply the principles of aggressive glycemic therapy (Cryer et al. 2003; Cryer 2008, 2010, 2011a; Rossetti et al. 2008; Amiel et al. 2008; Amiel 2009; Graveling and Frier 2009). 3) Consider the conventional risk factors (Chapter 4) (Table 4.1). 4) Consider the risk factors indicative of hypoglycemia-associated autonomic failure (HAAF) in diabetes (Chapter 4) (Table 4.1).

Acknowledge the problem

The issue of hypoglycemia should be addressed in every contact with sulfonylurea-, glinide-, or insulin-treated people with diabetes. Patient concerns about the reality, or even the possibility, of hypoglycemia can be a barrier to glycemic control (Gonder-Frederick et al. 2006; Nordfeldt and Ludvigsson 2005; Wild et al. 2007). Indeed, some studies suggest that people with insulin-treated diabetes are more concerned about the possibility of an episode of hypoglycemia than about the long-term complications of diabetes (Pramming et al. 1991; Nordfeldt and Ludvigsson 2005). Yet, patients are often reluctant to volunteer their concerns. They should be given the explicit opportunity to do so. It is also often helpful to question close associates of the patient, since they may have observed clues to episodes of hypoglycemia not recognized by the patient. Even if no concerns are expressed, examination of the self–plasma glucose monitoring record (or continuous glucose monitoring data) will often disclose that hypoglycemia is a problem.

Apply the principles of aggressive glycemic therapy

If hypoglycemia is a problem, each of the principles of aggressive glycemic therapy (Cryer et al. 2003; Cryer 2008, 2010, 2011a) (Table 6.1) should be considered and applied. Those of the author follow. They are generally consistent with those of others in the field (Rossetti et al. 2008; Amiel et al. 2008; Amiel 2009; Graveling and Frier 2009).

Patient education and empowerment are fundamentally important (Bendik et al. 2009; McIntyre et al. 2010; Keen et al. 2012). As the therapeutic regimen becomes progressively more

Table 6.1. Principles of Aggressive Glycemic Therapy of Diabetes

1.	Patient education and empowerment
2.	Frequent self–plasma glucose monitoring (and in some instances continuous glucose monitoring)
3.	Flexible and appropriate insulin (and other drug) regimens and use of diabetes treatment technologies
4.	Individualized glycemic goals
5.	Ongoing professional guidance and support

complex—early in type 1 diabetes and later in type 2 diabetes—the success of glycemic management becomes progressively more dependent on the many management decisions and the skills of the well-informed person with diabetes. Without those, it will often not be successful.

In addition to basic training about diabetes, people with sulfonylurea-, glinide-, or insulin-treated diabetes need to be taught about the anticipation, recognition, and treatment of hypoglycemia (Cox et al. 2004). They need to know how their medications can cause hypoglycemia. They need to know the common symptoms of hypoglycemia and, over time, to learn their individual most meaningful symptoms. They need to know how to treat (and not over-treat) hypoglycemia. Close associates, such as spouses, need to be taught how to recognize an episode of severe hypoglycemia and how to administer parenteral glucagon. Patients need to understand the conventional risk factors for hypoglycemia (Table 4.1), including the effects of the dose and timing of their individual secretagogue or insulin preparation(s) as well as the effects of missed meals and the overnight fast, alcohol, and exercise. With respect to the latter, they need strategies to defend against planned or unanticipated exercise. They also need to know that episodes of hypoglycemia (a risk factor for HAAF [Table 4.1]) signal an increased likelihood of future, often more severe, episodes. Indeed, Cox and colleagues have shown that increasingly frequent low self-monitored glucose levels identify an increasing risk of imminent severe hypoglycemia (Kovatchev et al. 1998, 2003; Cox et al. 2007). In a systematic analysis of prospectively obtained self–plasma glucose monitoring data and of the occurrence of severe hypoglycemia, they found that a recent increase in their calculated low blood glucose index detected ~60% of imminent (within 24 hours) episodes of severe hypoglycemia in both type 1 diabetes and insulin-treated type 2 diabetes (Cox et al. 2007). Finally, patients using continuous glucose monitoring need to learn how to apply those data to their attempts to minimize hypoglycemia as well as hyperglycemia. Again, the successful glycemic management of type 1 diabetes and of advanced type 2 diabetes is critically dependent on a well-informed person with diabetes.

It is reasonable to anticipate that frequent self–plasma glucose monitoring (supplemented in some instances by continuous glucose monitoring) will provide insight leading to rational modifications of the therapeutic regimen in individuals treated with insulin or with a sulfonylurea or a glinide. Logically, that would become more key to short-term management decisions as the regimen becomes more complex. Ideally, patients should monitor their plasma glucose level whenever they suspect hypoglycemia. That would not only confirm or deny hypoglycemia; it would also help the person learn the key symptoms of their hypoglycemic episodes and might lead to regimen adjustments. It is particularly important for people with hypoglycemia unawareness to monitor their plasma glucose level before performing a critical task such as driving.

Flexible and appropriate insulin (and other drug) regimens are clearly important. Treatment with insulin, a sulfonylurea, or a glinide can cause hypoglycemia in diabetes. Metformin, thiazolidinediones, α-glucosidase inhibitors, glucagon-like peptide-1 (GLP-1) receptor agonists, and dipeptidyl peptidase-IV (DPP-IV) inhibitors should not, and probably do not, cause hypoglycemia (Bolen et al. 2007; Phung et al. 2010; Tschope et al. 2011). That is true even for the GLP-1 receptor agonists and DPP-IV inhibitors, which are, among other mechanisms, insulin secretagogues. They produce glucose-dependent insulin secretion that disengages as plasma glucose concentrations fall into the normal range. However, the latter feature may be lost, and hypoglycemia can occur, when a GLP-1 receptor agonist or a DPP-IV inhibitor is used with a sulfonylurea (de Heer and Holst 2007). Indeed, all five categories of drugs increase the risk of hypoglycemia if used with insulin, a sulfonylurea, or a glinide. The bile acid sequestrant colesevelam and the dopamine receptor agonist bromocriptine (Gaziano et al. 2010; DeFronzo 2011) should not cause hypoglycemia. Among potential future glucose-lowering drug categories, agents that inhibit renal glucose re-absorption (Ferrannini et al. 2010) or activate G-protein coupled receptor 40 (Burant et al. 2012) should not cause hypoglycemia, while glucokinase activators might well cause hypoglycemia (Bonadonna et al. 2010; Matschinsky et al. 2011).

Although detimer and particularly glargine are longer acting than NPH insulin, with a half-time of approximately 24 hours, degludec is the most long-acting basal insulin (Heller et al. 2012; Garber et al. 2012). Sulfonylureas currently used widely—glyburide (glibenclamide), glimepiride, glipizide, and gliclazide—generally act within 24 hours. Glinides—repaglinide and nateglinide—are rapid-acting prandial glucose lowering drugs that are dosed with meals.

Among the commonly used sulfonylureas, glyburide [glibenclamide] is most often associated with hypoglycemia (Holstein and Egberts 2003; Gangji et al. 2007). In addition, high mortality has been reported in patients with diabetes and acute myocardial infarction who were treated with glyburide compared with those treated with glimepiride or gliclazide (Zeller et al. 2010). The use of a long-acting basal insulin analog (e.g., glargine or detimer), compared to NPH insulin, in a multiple daily injection (MDI) insulin regimen reduces at least the incidence of nocturnal hypoglycemia, perhaps that of total and symptomatic hypoglycemia, in type 1 diabetes and type 2 diabetes (Hirsch 2005; Horvath et al. 2007; Gough 2007; Monami et al. 2009; Little et al. 2011). Compared with glargine the use of the longer-acting basal analog degludec reduced confirmed nocturnal hypoglycemia in type 1 diabetes (Heller et al., 2012) and confirmed nocturnal and overall hypoglycemia in type 2 diabetes (Garber et al. 2012). Compared with human regular insulin, the use of a rapid-acting prandial insulin analog (e.g., lispro, aspart or glulisine) reduces the incidence of nocturnal hypoglycemia at least in type 1 diabetes (Hirsch 2005; Siebenhofer et al. 2006; Gough 2007). A basal–bolus MDI regimen— a basal long-acting insulin coupled with a prandial rapid-acting insulin as needed—has been reported to produce the lowest mean glycemia and rates of hypoglycemia compared with biphasic insulin twice daily or prandial insulin alone (Holman et al. 2009).

It seems likely that some, perhaps all, of the evolving diabetes treatment technologies—real-time continuous glucose monitoring (CGM), continuous subcutaneous insulin infusion (CSII), sensor-augmented CSII, and closed-loop insulin replacement—will ultimately be convincingly shown to be beneficial to patients with type 1 diabetes and those with advanced type 2 diabetes. That judgment will be based initially on compelling evidence that the technology improves glycemic control (typically, as assessed by A1C) without increasing the frequency or severity of hypoglycemia (or reduces hypoglycemia without deterioration of glycemic control) and the extent to which it does so. In short, is the technology clinically meaningful? Given that, issues such as the impact on quality of life and cost become relevant.

Real-time continuous glucose monitoring reports subcutaneous glucose concentrations, which lag changes in plasma glucose by ~15 minutes (as submitted), suffers from relative inaccuracy of the sensors at low glucose levels and, obviously, requires that the device be used (Raju 2006; Hermanides and De Vries 2010). Nonetheless, use of real-time CGM has been found to be associated with an A1C reduction in the range of 0.4–0.6% in adults with type 1 diabetes who generally actually used the device (Juvenile Diabetes Research Foundation [JDRF] Continuous Glucose Monitoring Study Group 2008, 2009a, 2009b, 2010) without an increase in detected hypoglycemia. However, the fact that the trials were underpowered to detect an increase in hypoglycemia was acknowledged (JDRF 2008). In another study of patients with type 1 diabetes the total number of subcutaneous glucose excursions to <63 mg/dl (3.5 mmol/l) tended to be reduced and those during the night were reduced significantly during continuous glucose monitoring (Battelino et al. 2011); mean A1C levels were 0.3% lower in that group. Interestingly, real-time CGM was found to result in increased epinephrine secretory responses to hypoglycemia, i.e., was found to partially reverse HAAF, presumably the result of less iatrogenic hypoglycemia although that was not documented, in patients with type 1 diabetes (Ly et al. 2011). Sensor-augmented pump therapy – the combination of real-time CGM with CSII—has been reported to achieve an ~0.5% greater decrease in A1C than MDI alone without an increase in hypoglycemia in a one year study (Bergenstal et al. 2010). A sensor-augmented CSII pump that temporarily suspends insulin infusion when the CGM value falls below a pre-selected value (a low glucose suspend, or LGS, feature) has been reported to reduce CGM excursions below 70 mg/dl (3.9 mmol/l) by ~25% in patients with type 1 diabetes although the sequential experimental design—no LGS, then LGS—may have compromised interpretation of the data (Danne et al. 2011). In an exercise study LGS on (at a CGM value of 70 mg/dl) compared with LGS off hardly blunted the mean nadir plasma glucose concentration (60 vs. 58 mg/dl) (Garg 2012) and in a nocturnal study LGS was shown to result in hyperglycemia the following morning (Ly et al. 2012). Nonetheless, CGM has not been shown to prevent severe hypoglycemia (Hermanides et al. 2011; Langendam et al. 2012; Yeh et al. 2012).

Continuous subcutaneous insulin infusion (CSII), typically with a rapid-acting insulin analog, should be superior to multiple daily insulin injection (MDI), typically with a long-acting basal insulin analog and a rapid-acting prandial insulin analog, because CSII permits variation in basal insulin infusion across the day. Several meta-analyses have led to the conclusion that CSII results in slightly better glycemic control, with A1C values lower by ~0.2–0.4%, without an increase in hypoglycemia in adults and children with type 1 diabetes (Jeitler et al. 2008; Fatourechi et al. 2009; Pankowska et al. 2009; Langendam et al. 2012; Yeh et al. 2012). However, these meta-analyses included a variety of trials. One randomized controlled trial comparing CSII with an insulin analog and MDI with basal and preprandial insulin analogs found no difference in achieved A1C or in the prevalence of hypoglycemia (Bolli et al. 2009). Notably, CSII was 3.9 times more expensive. A systemic review of eight trials comparing CSII with insulin analog–based MDI came to the same conclusion (Cummins et al. 2010). A systematic review of six randomized controlled trials in pregnant women with diabetes did not show a significant difference between CSII and MDI (Mukhopadhyay et al. 2007).

Based on a systematic review and meta-analysis of randomized controlled trials published up to 2012, Yeh et al. (2012) concluded that CSII (compared with MDI), real-time CGM (compared with SMPG), and sensor-augmented CSII (compared with MDI and SMPG) had not been shown to reduce the incidence of severe hypoglycemia in type 1 or type 2 diabetes. However, the authors pointed out the limitations of the available data, including generally small sample sizes and relatively short study durations, limited study of young children and older adults, variable study quality, and variable definitions of hypoglycemia. Furthermore, there was slightly greater reduction of A1C with CSII in type 1 diabetes and larger reductions in A1C with real-time CGM and with sensor-augmented CSII. Thus, these technologies may, or may not, be shown to reduce the frequency of hypoglycemia in the future.

Clearly, flawless closed-loop insulin replacement would solve the problem of hypoglycemia in diabetes. The challenge of closed-loop insulin replacement (Wilinska et al. 2009; Hovorka et al. 2010; Hovorka et al. 2011; Murphy et al. 2011), and even closed-loop bihormonal (insulin and glucagon) replacement (El-Khatib et al. 2010; Castle et al. 2010) is being addressed. The overnight period has been an initial focus since that does not require the system to include meal-stimulated insulin replacement.

A consistent observation since the DCCT (1991, 1993, 1997) is that more than half of the episodes of hypoglycemia, including severe hypoglycemia, occur during the night (Chico et al. 2003; Guillod et al. 2007). That is typically the longest interval between meals and between self–plasma glucose monitoring and includes the time of maximal sensitivity to insulin. In addition to the use of insulin analogs (Hirsch 2005; Horvath et al. 2007; Gough 2007) or closed-loop insulin replacement (Wilinska et al. 2009), approaches to the prevention of nocturnal hypoglycemia include attempts to produce sustained delivery of exogenous carbohydrate or sustained endogenous glucose production throughout the night (Raju 2006). With respect to the former approach, a conventional bedtime snack or bedtime administration of uncooked cornstarch has not been found to be effective (Raju et al. 2006); the duration of their glycemic action is too short. With respect to the latter approach, bedtime administration of 5.0 mg of the epinephrine-simulating β_2-adrenergic agonist terbutaline has been shown to prevent nocturnal hypoglycemia in adults with aggressively treated type 1 diabetes, albeit at the expense of hyperglycemia the following morning (Raju et al. 2006). A 2.5 mg bedtime dose of terbutaline produced intermediate results on nocturnal plasma glucose levels without morning hyperglycemia (Cooperberg et al. 2008). The higher plasma glucose concentrations following administration of terbutaline were likely the result of β_2-adrenergic stimulation of hepatic and renal glucose production, but may also have been the result of β_2-adrenergic stimulation at a ventromedial hypothalamic site with subsequent sympathoadrenal, at least adrenomedullary, epinephrine, and α-cell glucagon secretion (Szepietowska et al. 2011). An alternative approach in patients using CSII is to reduce the basal insulin infusion dose at bedtime. A comparison of 1) a 20% reduction in insulin dose at bedtime, 2) a 2.5 mg dose of terbutaline at bedtime, and 3) no treatment at bedtime in children with type 1 diabetes disclosed that the reduction in insulin dose and terbutaline administration resulted in comparable hyperglycemia during the night but terbutaline more consistently prevented nocturnal hypoglycemia (Taplin et al. 2010). An insulin infusion pump with a glucose–monitor signaled two-hour low glucose suspend feature has been tested (Choudhary 2011). Obviously, these, and other potentially effective treatments, which have been reviewed (Cryer 2011b), will need to be tested in suitably powered, randomized controlled trials if they are to be used to prevent hypoglycemia. Nocturnal hypoglycemia is also a reasonable initial target for closed-loop insulin replacement (Wilinska et al. 2009; Hovorka et al. 2010). Parenthetically, there is now considerable evidence against the Somogyi hypothesis (Guillod et al. 2007); morning hyperglycemia is the result of insulin lack, not post-hypoglycemic insulin resistance (Havlin and Cryer 1987; Tordjman et al. 1987; Hirsch et al. 1990). There is a dawn phenomenon—a growth hormone–mediated increase in the nighttime to morning plasma glucose concentration (Campbell et al. 1985)—but its magnitude is small (Periello et al. 1991).

Other special conditions relevant to hypoglycemia include the elderly, drivers, and pregnant women. Glucose counterregulatory defenses against falling plasma glucose concentrations are impaired minimally by age per se (Marker et al. 1992; Meneilly et al. 1994). Nonetheless, diabetes is increasingly common in older individuals and that includes the transition of type 2 diabetes to absolute endogenous insulin deficiency and all of the resulting pathophysiology (Chapter 3) and risk factors for hypoglycemia (Chapter 4) discussed earlier. In addition to HAAF, issues such as co-morbidities including renal insufficiency, polypharmacy, and impaired cognition are more often relevant in older individuals (Alagiakrishnan and Mereu 2010). Also, the issue of relative benefit from glycemic control comes into play. It is difficult to separate effects of age from those of duration of diabetes. For example, although older individuals with type 2 diabetes had less intense symptoms during hypoglycemia than middle-aged patients, they also had known diabetes for more than twice as long (Bremer et al. 2009).

Drivers with a history of recurrent hypoglycemia-related driving mishaps have been found to have more symptoms during euglycemia (i.e., more symptom "noise"), greater driving-simulator impairments, and less intense hormonal counterregulatory responses to hypoglycemia (Cox et al. 2010). Obviously, self-monitoring of plasma glucose is critical prior to performance of any critical task, such as driving, particularly for individuals with hypoglycemia unawareness. Finally, up to 45% of pregnant women with type 1 diabetes experience severe hypoglycemia, with substantially higher rates in the first trimester (Nielsen et al. 2008). There is some evidence that pregnancy is associated with suppression of glucose counterregulation (Rosenn et al. 1996).

A reasonable individualized glycemic goal is the lowest A1C that does not cause severe hypoglycemia (that requiring the assistance of another person), preserves awareness of hypoglycemia, and causes, at worst, an acceptable number of documented episodes of symptomatic hypoglycemia at a given stage in the evolution of the individual's diabetes (Cryer 2011b). It would seem that the selection of such an individualized glycemic goal should rest largely on the required therapy and the relative risk of iatrogenic hypoglycemia. During effective therapy of early type 2 diabetes with lifestyle changes or with pharmacological glucose-lowering therapy other than a sulfonylurea, a glinide, or insulin, a reasonable glycemic goal might be a normal A1C. That might be beneficial over a substantial portion of the course of type 2 diabetes. But, such therapies are seldom successful over a lifetime of type 2 diabetes and are not effective in type 1 diabetes. During therapy of type 2 diabetes with a sulfonylurea, a glinide, or insulin or of type 1 diabetes with insulin, the glycemic goal might be an A1C of <7% (ADA 2012). That sometimes can be accomplished safely relatively early in type 2 diabetes—even shortly after oral agent failure (UK Hypo Group 2007)—or very shortly after diagnosis in type 1 diabetes. But, it is often not possible later. If an A1C <7% is not achievable safely, there is demonstrable benefit from reducing A1C from high to lower, albeit still above optimal, levels (DCCT 1995; Lachin et al. 2008). Indeed, a mean A1C of 7.5% was associated with an all-cause mortality risk ratio of 1.0 in the U.K. General Practice Research Database (Currie et al. 2010). Finally, glucose levels low enough to prevent symptoms of hyperglycemia become a reasonable glycemic goal in individuals with a limited life expectancy or functional capacity in whom glycemic control is unlikely to be beneficial.

Aggressive treatment of patients with stress hyperglycemia or diabetes in intensive care units to normoglycemia (e.g., plasma glucose concentrations of 80–110 mg/dl [4.4–6.1 mmol/l]) has not been found to produce consistent benefits, increases the risk of hypoglycemia, and may increase mortality (NICE-SUGAR 2009; Kavanagh and McCowen 2010; Kansagara et al. 2011). A higher glycemic goal, perhaps 140–180 mg/dl (7.8–10.0 mmol/l), is reasonable (Moghissi et al. 2009).

Finally, because the glycemic management of diabetes is empirical, caregivers should provide ongoing professional guidance and support and work with the individual patient over time to find the best method of glycemic control at a given time in the course of that patient's diabetes. Care is best accomplished by a team that includes, in addition to a physician, professionals trained in, and dedicated to, translating the standards of care (ADA 2012) into the care of individual patients and making full use of modern communication and computing technologies.

Because this is a book on hypoglycemia in diabetes, the therapeutic discussion is focused on glycemic control. Obviously, that is only part of the appropriate treatment. Diet and exercise leading to weight loss, blood pressure and blood lipid control, and smoking cessation are also fundamentally important in many people with diabetes (Gaede et al. 2003).

Consider the conventional risk factors

In a patient with iatrogenic hypoglycemia, each of the conventional risk factors, those that result in relative or absolute insulin excess (Table 4.1), should be considered carefully, and the therapeutic regimen should be adjusted appropriately. In addition to the dose, type, and timing of insulin or insulin secretagogue medications, those risk factors include conditions in which exogenous glucose delivery or endogenous glucose production is decreased, glucose utilization or sensitivity to insulin is increased, or insulin clearance is reduced.

Consider the risk factors indicative of HAAF

Risk factors indicative of HAAF include the degree of absolute endogenous insulin deficiency, a history of severe hypoglycemia or hypoglycemia unawareness or both, as well as any relationship between hypoglycemic episodes and recent antecedent hypoglycemia, prior exercise, or sleep, and lower A1C levels (Table 4.1). Unless the cause is easily remediable, a history of severe hypoglycemia should prompt consideration of a fundamental regimen adjustment. Without that, the risk of a subsequent episode of severe hypoglycemia is high (Kovatchev et al. 1998, 2003; Cox et al. 2007; DCCT 1997). Given a history of hypoglycemia unawareness, a 2- to 3-week period of scrupulous avoidance of hypoglycemia, which may require acceptance of somewhat higher glycemic goals in the short term, is advisable, since that can be expected to restore awareness (Fanelli et al. 1993, 1994b; Cranston et al. 1994; Dagogo-Jack et al. 1994). A history of late post-exercise hypoglycemia, nocturnal hypoglycemia, or both should prompt appropriately timed regimen adjustments (generically, less insulin action, more carbohydrate ingestion, or both) or, failing these, a pharmacological treatment (Raju et al. 2006).

To date, the only established approach to reversal of hypoglycemia unawareness, and at least in part the attenuated epinephrine component of defective glucose counterregulation, is a period of scrupulous avoidance of hypoglycemia (Fanelli et al. 1993, 1994b; Cranston et al. 1994; Dagogo-Jack et al. 1994). Reversal of the attenuated sympathoadrenal response would correct the key feature of HAAF and therefore reduce the risk of hypoglycemia. Potential future approaches to the problem have been reviewed (Cryer 2011b) and were summarized earlier (Chapter 4). Successful islet or pancreas transplantation largely reverses the key features of HAAF (Rickels 2012).

TREATMENT OF HYPOGLYCEMIA

Hypoglycemia causes functional brain failure that is corrected in the vast majority of instances after the plasma glucose concentration is raised (Cryer 2007). Profound, prolonged hypoglycemia can cause brain death but most fatal episodes are the result of other mechanisms, presumably ventricular arrhythmias (Chapter 3). Clearly, the plasma glucose concentration should be raised to normal levels promptly. Data from a rodent model of extreme hypoglycemia suggest that post-treatment glycemia contributes to neuronal death (Suh et al. 2007). Although the clinical extrapolation of that finding is unclear (Cryer 2007), it may be that post-hypoglycemia hyperglycemia should be avoided, at least after an episode of profound, prolonged hypoglycemia.

In people with diabetes, most episodes of asymptomatic hypoglycemia (detected by self–plasma glucose monitoring or continuous glucose monitoring) or of mild-moderate symptomatic hypoglycemia are effectively self-treated by ingestion of glucose tablets or carbohydrate-containing juice, soft drinks, candy, other snacks, or a meal (Cryer 2008; MacCuish 1993; Wiethop and Cryer 1993a). A reasonable dose is 20 g of glucose (Cryer 2008; Wiethop and Cryer 1993a) (Figure 6.1). Clinical improvement should occur in 15–20 minutes. However, in the setting of ongoing hyperinsulinemia, the glycemic response to oral glucose is transient—typically <2 hours (Wiethop and Cryer 1993a). Thus, ingestion of a more substantial snack or meal shortly after the plasma glucose level is raised is generally advisable. In contrast to swallowed glucose, glucose applied to the buccal mucosa is not absorbed (Gunning and Garber 1978). Administration of the somatostatin analog octreotide, which inhibits insulin secretion, can be used as a supplement to glucose administration in the treatment of sulfonylurea-induced hypoglycemia (Boyle et al. 1993; Dougherty and Klein-Schwartz 2010).

Parenteral treatment is required when a hypoglycemic

patient is unwilling (because of neuroglycopenia) or unable to take carbohydrate orally. Glucagon, injected subcutaneously or intramuscularly in a usual dose of 1.0 mg in adults by an associate of the patient, is often used. That can be lifesaving, but it often causes substantial, albeit transient, hyperglycemia (Figure 6.1), and it can cause nausea or even vomiting. Smaller doses of glucagon (e.g., 150 µg), repeated if necessary, have been found to be effective without side effects in children (Haymond and Schreiner 2001). Because it stimulates insulin secretion, glucagon might be less useful in patients other than those with type 1 diabetes or advanced type 2 diabetes. Indeed, glucagon has been reported to cause hypoglycemia in nondiabetic individuals (Murad et al. 2009; Cryer et al. 2009). Because it acts primarily by stimulating hepatic glycogenolysis, glucagon

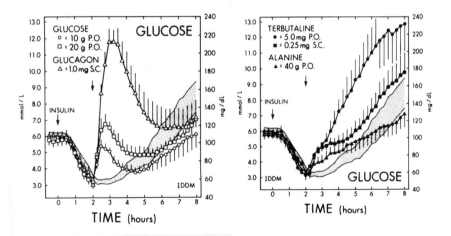

Figure 6.1. Mean (±SE) plasma glucose concentrations during insulin-induced hypoglycemia in patients with type 1 diabetes (IDDM) in the absence of an intervention (shaded area) and after the indicated interventions. S.C., subcutaneous, P.O., per os. From Wiethop and Cryer 1993b, reproduced with permission of the American Diabetes Association.

treatment is ineffective in glycogen-depleted individuals (e.g., after a binge of alcohol ingestion).

Although glucagon can be administered intravenously by medical personnel, in that setting intravenous glucose is the standard parenteral therapy. A common initial dose of intravenous glucose is 25 g (Cryer 2008; MacCuish 1993); lower doses could be used in a setting in which plasma glucose concentrations can be measured serially. The glycemic response to intravenous glucose is of course transient in the setting of ongoing hyperinsulinemia. A subsequent glucose infusion is often needed, and food should be provided as soon as the patient is able to ingest it safely.

The duration of a hypoglycemic episode is a function of its cause. An episode caused by a rapid-acting insulin secretagogue or insulin analog will be relatively brief, and that caused by a long-acting insulin analog will be substantially longer. A sulfonylurea overdose, or that of a long-acting insulin analog, can result in prolonged hypoglycemia requiring hospitalization.

CLINICAL PRACTICE GUIDELINES

Many of the principles discussed in this book were incorporated, by a panel organized by The Endocrine Society, into a set of clinical practice guidelines for the evaluation and management of adult hypoglycemic disorders (Cryer et al. 2009). The development of the guidelines included an assessment of the strength of the supporting evidence, resulting in suggestions based on weaker evidence and recommendations based on stronger evidence. The suggestions and recommendations concerning hypoglycemia in people with diabetes are listed in Table 6.2.

Table 6.2. Clinical Practice Guidelines (Cryer et al. 2009)

1. We suggest that individuals with diabetes become concerned about the possibility of developing hypoglycemia when the self-monitored blood glucose concentration is falling rapidly or is <70 mg/dl (<3.9 mmol/l).

2. Given the established long-term microvascular, and potential macro-vascular, benefits of glycemic control, we recommend that the thera-peutic glycemic goal be the lowest mean glycemia (e.g., A1C) that can be accomplished safely in a given patient at a given point in the pro-gression of that individual patient's diabetes.

3. We recommend that the prevention of hypoglycemia in diabetes involves addressing the issue in each patient contact and, if hypoglyce-mia is a problem, making adjustments in the regimen based on review and application of the principles of aggressive glycemic therapy—patient education and empowerment, frequent self–blood glucose monitoring, flexible and appropriate insulin or insulin secretagogue regimens, individualized glycemic goals, and ongoing professional guidance and support—and consideration of each of the known risk factors for hypoglycemia.

4. We recommend that both the conventional risk factors and those indicative of compromised defenses against hypoglycemia be consid-ered in a patient with recurrent treatment-induced hypoglycemia. The conventional risk factors are excessive or ill-timed dosing of, or wrong type of, insulin or insulin secretagogue and conditions under which exogenous glucose delivery or endogenous glucose production is decreased, glucose utilization is increased, sensitivity to insulin is increased, or insulin clearance is decreased. Compromised defenses against hypoglycemia are indicated by the degree of endogenous insulin deficiency, a history of severe hypoglycemia or hypoglycemia unawareness or both, as well as recent antecedent hypoglycemia, prior exercise or sleep, and lower glycemic goals per se.

5. With a history of hypoglycemia unawareness (i.e., recurrent hypogly-cemia without symptoms), we recommend a 2- to 3-week period of scrupulous avoidance of hypoglycemia, with the anticipation that awareness of hypoglycemia will return in many patients

6. Unless the cause is easily remediable, we recommend that an episode of severe hypoglycemia should lead to a fundamental review of the treatment regimen.

7. We recommend that urgent treatment of hypoglycemia should be accomplished by ingestion of carbohydrates if that is feasible and by parenteral glucagon or glucose if the former is not feasible.

Chapter 7.
Perspective on Hypoglycemia in Diabetes

D iabetes is an increasingly common chronic disease. Its human and economic costs are large and, despite advances in therapy, are growing because of the increasing prevalence of diabetes. Since the introduction of insulin therapy in 1922, it has been possible to prevent early death from diabetic ketoacidosis or hyperosmolar coma and to eliminate symptoms of uncontrolled hyperglycemia in the vast majority of patients. However, by the mid-20th century it was apparent that the early insulin therapies did not prevent the long-term microvascular and macrovascular complications of diabetes. Diabetes became the leading cause of end-stage renal disease requiring dialysis or transplantation, of blindness with its onset in working-age adults, and of nontraumatic amputations, and most people with diabetes died from cardiovascular disease. There were important practical advances in diabetes care in the late 20th century. Those included the development of A1C measurements to quantitate overall glycemic control, self–plasma glucose monitoring (and more recently, continuous glucose monitoring) to assess short-term glycemic control, insulin analogs with more favorable (albeit less than ideal) pharmacokinetic profiles, an array of new drugs that lower plasma glucose concentrations early in the course of type 2 diabetes, and the concept of a diabetes care team, among others. Since the landmark Diabetes Control and Complications Trial in type 1 diabetes, published in 1993, many studies, including the U.K. Prospective Diabetes Study in type 2 diabetes, have led to widespread consensus that long-term glycemic control prevents or delays at least the microvascular complications of diabetes. Nonetheless, microvascular and macrovascular complications are still a reality for many people with diabetes. Furthermore, the impact of the barrier of iatrogenic hypoglycemia, the limiting factor in the glycemic management of many people with diabetes, has been more widely appreciated (Chapter 1).

Glycemic control, which is the focus of this book because its topic is hypoglycemia in diabetes, is but one aspect of the management of diabetes. For example, it is now clear that blood lipid and blood pressure control, as well as blood glucose control, are fundamentally important to the prevention or delay of the vascular complications of diabetes. However, while it is now possible to drive LDL cholesterol to subphysiological levels and to normalize blood pressure pharmacologically, usually without major side effects, in most people with diabetes, it is still not possible to maintain euglycemia over a lifetime of diabetes in the vast majority of patients because of the barrier of iatrogenic hypoglycemia. Weight reduction and smoking cessation are often additional relevant challenges.

Based on insight into the physiology of glucose counterregulation (Chapter 2) and its pathophysiology, and the relationship of the latter to clinical hypoglycemia, in diabetes (Chapter 3), many risk factors for iatrogenic hypoglycemia have been identified (Chapter 4) and a working definition and classification of hypoglycemia in diabetes has been proposed (Chapter 5). Thus, it is now possible to both improve glycemic control and reduce the risk of hypoglycemia in many people with diabetes (Chapter 6).

It is important for both diabetes caregivers and people with diabetes to keep the problem of iatrogenic hypoglycemia in perspective. The underlying principle of the glycemic management of diabetes is that maintenance of glycemia as close to the nondiabetic range as can be accomplished safely over time is in the patient's best interests. It reduces the development of microvascular complications and may reduce that of macrovascular complications. The extent to which that goal can be met is a function of many factors, including the type of diabetes and the stage in the evolution of diabetes in an individual patient. Type 2 diabetes is, by far, the more common type of diabetes. Early in the course of type 2 diabetes, hyperglycemia may respond to lifestyle changes, specifically weight loss, or to plasma glucose–lowering drugs that do not raise circulating insulin levels and therefore should not, and probably do not, cause hypoglycemia. Those include the biguanide metformin, thiazolidinediones, and α-glucosidase inhibitors that do not cause hyperinsulinemia. They also include GLP-1 receptor agonists and dipeptidyl peptidase-IV (DPP-IV) inhibitors, which raise insulin levels only in the presence of hyperglycemia. In theory, when such drugs are effective, there is no reason not to accelerate their dosing until euglycemia is achieved in the absence of nonglycemic side effects. The reality, however, is that either initially, or over time, as patients with type 2 diabetes become progressively more insulin deficient, these drugs (even in combination) fail to provide glycemic control. Insulin secretagogues, a sulfonylurea or a glinide, are also effective early in the course of type 2 diabetes, although these raise endogenous insulin levels and therefore introduce the possibility of iatrogenic hypoglycemia. Nonetheless, as emphasized in Chapter 1, the frequency of iatrogenic hypoglycemia is relatively low (at least with current glycemic goals) during treatment with an insulin secretagogue, or even with insulin, early in the course of type 2 diabetes when glucose counterregulatory defenses are intact. Thus, over most of the course of the most common type of diabetes, it is possible to achieve a meaningful degree of glycemic control with no risk or relatively low risk of iatrogenic hypoglycemia. Clearly, that is beneficial to those patients. Therefore, it is fundamentally important that concerns about the risk of hypoglycemia should not be used as an excuse for poor glycemic control by diabetes caregivers or by people with diabetes in most instances. Rather, both should strive to achieve and maintain the greatest glycemic control that can be accomplished safely in a given patient with diabetes at a given stage of his or her diabetes.

All people with type 1 diabetes, and ultimately most with type 2 diabetes, require treatment with insulin. Insulin is demonstrably effective. Given in sufficient doses, it will lower plasma glucose concentrations in virtually all people with diabetes. Insulin therapy is life-saving in type 1 diabetes and is necessary in those with advanced (i.e., absolutely insulin deficient) type 2 diabetes. In the latter patients, it should be introduced earlier, rather than later, when other therapies fail to achieve glycemic control. The difficulty of course is that, while it is demonstrably effective, insulin is not demonstrably safe. Because of the pharmacokinetic imperfections of insulin therapy, particularly in the setting of compromised glucose counterregulation (the syndromes of defective glucose counterregulation and hypoglycemia unawareness and therefore hypoglycemia-associated autonomic failure) that develops early in type 1 diabetes and later in type 2 diabetes, it is limited by the barrier of iatrogenic hypoglycemia. Therefore, the goal of long-term euglycemia is not feasible in such patients with current insulin regimens.

Although it can be minimized in many patients, the problem of iatrogenic hypoglycemia in type 1 diabetes and advanced type 2 diabetes has not been solved. Diabetes will someday be cured and prevented, but no one knows when that will be accomplished. Short of that, elimination of hypoglycemia from the lives of people with diabetes will likely be accomplished by the development of methods that provide plasma glucose–regulated insulin replacement (i.e., closed-loop insulin therapy) or secretion (i.e., implantation of insulin-secreting cells or expansion of β-cell mass). In the meantime, innovative research, ranging from studies of the fundamental molecular and cellular mechanisms of the physiology and pathophysiology of glucose counterregulation to clinical trials of novel approaches to the prevention of iatrogenic hypoglycemia, is clearly needed if we are to improve the lives of all people affected by diabetes by eliminating hypoglycemia.

Bibliography

Abraira C, Colwell JA, Nuttall FQ, Swain CT, Nagel NJ, Comstock JP, Emanuele NV, Levin SR, Henderson W, Lee HS. 1995. Veterans Affairs cooperative study on glycemic control and complications in type II diabetes (VA CSCM). *Diabetes Care* 18:1113–1123.

Action to Control Cardiovascular Risk in Diabetes Study Group [ACCORD]. 2008. Effects of intensive glucose lowering in type 2 diabetes. *N Engl J Med* 358:2545–2559.

———. 2011. Long-term effects of intensive glucose lowering on cardiovascular outcomes. *N Engl J Med* 364:818–828.

Adler GK, Bonyhay I, Failing H, Waring E, Dotson S, Freeman R. 2009. Antecedent hypoglycemia impairs cardiovascular function. Implications for rigorous glycemic control. *Diabetes* 58:360–366.

ADVANCE Collaborative Group [ADVANCE]. 2008. Intensive blood glucose control and vascular outcomes in patients with type 2 diabetes. *N Engl J Med* 358:2560–2572.

Akram K, Pedersen-Bjergaard U, Carstensen B, Borch-Johnsen K, Thorsteinsson B. 2006. Frequency and risk factors for severe hypoglycaemia in insulin-treated type 2 diabetes: a cross sectional survey. *Diabet Med* 23:750–756.

————. 2009. Prospective and retrospective recording of severe hypoglycaemia, and assessment of hypoglycaemia awareness in insulin-treated type 2 diabetes. *Diabet Med* 26:1306–1308.

Al-Noori S, Sanders NM, Taborsky GJ Jr, Wilkinson CW, Zavosh A, West C, Sanders CM, Figlewicz DP. 2008. Recurrent hypoglycemia alters hypothalamic expression of the regulatory proteins FosB and synaptophysin. *Am J Physiol Regul Integr Comp Physiol* 295:R1446–R1454.

Alagiakrishnan K, Mereu L. 2010. Approach to managing hypoglycemia in elderly patients with diabetes. *Postgrad Med* 122:129–137.

Allen C, LeCaire T, Palta M, Daniels K, Meredith M, D'Alessio DJ, for the Wisconsin Diabetes Registry Project. 2001. Risk factors for frequent and severe hypoglycemia in type 1 diabetes. *Diabetes Care* 24:1878–1881.

American Diabetes Association [ADA]. 2012. Standards of medical care in diabetes. *Diabetes Care* 34(Suppl. 1):S11–S63.

American Diabetes Association Workgroup on Hypoglycemia. 2005. Defining and reporting hypoglycemia in diabetes. *Diabetes Care* 28:1245–1249.

Amiel SA. 2009. Hypoglycemia: from the laboratory to the clinic. *Diabetes Care* 32:1364–1371.

Amiel SA, Dixon T, Mann R, Jameson K. 2008. Hypoglycaemia in type 2 diabetes. *Diabet Med* 25:245–254.

Amiel SA, Sherwin RS, Simonson DC, Tamborlane WV. 1988. Effect of intensive insulin therapy on glycemic thresholds for counterregulatory hormone release. *Diabetes* 37:901–907.

Arbeláez AM, Powers WJ, Videen TO, Price JL, Cryer PE. 2008. Attenuation of counterregulatory responses to recurrent hypoglycemia by active thalamic inhibition. A mechanism for hypoglycemia-associated autonomic failure. *Diabetes* 57:470–475.

Arbeláez AM, Rutlin JR, Hershey TG, Powers WJ, Videen TO, Cryer PE. 2012. Thalamic activation during slightly subphysiological glycemia in humans. *Diabetes Care* 2012. [Epub ahead of print]

Arbeláez AM, Tsalikian E, Mauras N, Wilson DM, Tamborlane WV, Sherr JL, Xing D, Kollman C, Ruedy K, Cryer PE, White NH, Diabetes Research in Children Network (DirecNet). 2012. Counterregulatory hormone responses in youth with short duration of type 1 diabetes (abstract). *Diabetes* 61:A320.

Åsvold BO, Sand T, Hestad K, Bjørgaas MR. 2010. Cognitive function in type 1 diabetic adults with early exposure to severe hypoglycemia. A 16-year follow-up study. *Diabetes Care* 33:1945–1947.

Auer RN. 1986. Progress review: hypoglycemic brain damage. *Stroke* 17:699–708.

Aung PP, Strachan MWJ, Frier BM, Butcher I, Deary IJ, Price JF on behalf of the Edinburgh Type 2 Diabetes Study Investigators. 2012. Severe hypoglycaemia and late-life cognitive ability in older people with type 2 diabetes: the Edinburgh Type 2 Diabetes Study. *Diabet Med* 29:328–336.

Banarer S, Cryer PE. 2003. Sleep-related hypoglycemia-associated autonomic failure in type 1 diabetes. Reduced awakening from sleep during hypoglycemia. *Diabetes* 52:1195–1203.

Banarer S, McGregor VP, Cryer PE. 2002. Intraislet hyperinsulinemia prevents the glucagon response to hypoglycemia despite an intact autonomic response. *Diabetes* 51:958–965.

Bao S, Briscoe VJ, Tate DB, Davis SN. 2009. Effects of differing antecedent increases of plasma cortisol on counterregulatory responses during subsequent exercise in type 1 diabetes. *Diabetes* 58:2100–2108.

Battelino T, Phillip M, Bratina N, Nimri R, Oskarsson P, Bolinder J. 2011. Effect of continuous glucose monitoring on hypoglycemia in type 1 diabetes. *Diabetes Care* 34:795–800.

Beléndez M, Hernández-Mijares A. 2009. Beliefs about insulin as a predictor of fear of hypoglycaemia. *Chronic Illn* 5:250–256.

Bell D, Huddart A, Krebs J. 2010. Driving and insulin-treated diabetes: comparing practices in Scotland and New Zealand. *Diabet Med* 27:1093–1095.

Ben Salem C, Fathallah N, Hmouda H, Bouraoui K. 2011. Drug-induced hypoglycaemia: an update. *Drug Saf* 34:21–45.

Bendik CF, Keller U, Moriconi N, Gessler A, Schindler Ch, Zulewski H, Ruiz J, Puder JJ. 2009. Training in flexible intensive insulin therapy improves quality of life, decreases the risk of hypoglycaemia and ameliorates poor metabolic control in patients with type 1 diabetes. *Diabetes Res Clin Pract* 83:327–333.

Benedict C, Hallschmid M, Hatke A, Schultes B, Fehm HL, Born J, Kern W. 2004. Intranasal insulin improves memory in humans. *Psychoneuroendocrinology* 29:1326–1334.

Benedict C, Hallschmid M, Schultes B, Born J. 2007. Intranasal insulin to improve memory function in humans. *Neuroendocrinology* 86:136–142.

Benedict L, Nelson CA, Schunk E, Sullwold K, Seaquist ER. 2006. Effect of insulin on the brain activity obtained during visual and memory tasks in healthy human subjects. *Neuroendocrinology* 83:20–26.

Bennett WL, Maruthur NM, Singh S, Segal JB, Wilson LM, Chatterjee R, Marinopoulos SS, Puhan MA, Ranasinghe P, Block L, Nicholson WK, Hutfless S, Bass EB, Bolen S. 2011. Comparative effectiveness and safety of medications for type 2 diabetes: an update including new drugs and 2-drug combinations. *Ann Intern Med* 154:602–613.

Bergenstal RM, Tamborlane WV, Ahmann A, Buse JB, Dailey G, Davis SN, Joyce C, Peoples T, Perkins BA, Welsh JB, Willi SM, Wood MA, for the STAR 3 Study Group. 2010. Effectiveness of sensor-augmented insulin-pump therapy in type 1 diabetes. *N Engl J Med* 363:311–320.

Berger B, Stenström G, Sundkvist G. 2000. Random C-peptide in the classification of diabetes. Scand J Clin *Lab Invest* 60:687–694.

Bergman RN. 2007. Orchestration of glucose homeostasis. *Diabetes* 56:1489–1501.

Berk MA, Clutter WE, Skor D, Shah SD, Gingerich RP, Parvin CA, Cryer PE. 1985. Enhanced glycemic responsiveness to epinephrine in insulin-dependent diabetes mellitus is the result of the inability to secrete insulin. *J Clin Invest* 75:1842–1851.

Berlin I, Grimaldi A, Payan C, Sachon C, Bosquet F, Thervet F, Puech AJ. 1987. Hypoglycemic symptoms and decreased β-adrenergic sensitivity in insulin dependent diabetic patients. *Diabetes Care* 10:742–747.

Bhatnagar S, Huber R, Nowak N, Trotter P. 2002. Lesions of the posterior paraventricular thalamus block habituation of hypothalamic-pituitary-adrenal responses to repeated restraint. *J Neuroendocrinol* 14:403–410.

Bhatnagar S, Viau V, Chu A, Soriano L, Meijer OC, Dallman MF. 2000. A cholecystokinin-mediated pathway to the paraventricular thalamus is recruited in chronically stressed rats and regulates hypothalamic-pituitary-adrenal function. *J Neurosci* 20:5564–5573.

Biessels GJ, Deary IJ, Ryan CM. 2008. Cognition and diabetes: a lifespan perspective. *Lancet Neurol* 7:184–190.

Bingham EM, Dunn JT, Smith D, Sutcliffe-Goulden J, Reed LJ, Marsden PK, Amiel SA. 2005. Differential changes in brain glucose metabolism during hypoglycaemia accompany loss of hypoglycaemia awareness in men with type 1 diabetes mellitus. An [11C]3-O-methylDglucose PET study. *Diabetologia* 48:2080-2089.

Bingham EM, Hopkins D, Smith D, Pernet A, Hallet W, Reed L, Marsden PK, Amiel SA. 2002. The role of insulin in human brain glucose metabolism. An [18]fluoro-deoxyglucose positron emission tomography study. *Diabetes* 51:3384–3390.

Blasetti A, Chiuri RM, Tocco AM, Di Giulio CD, Mattei PA, Ballone E, Chiarelli F, Verrotti A. 2011. The effect of recurrent severe hypoglycemia on cognitive performance in children with type 1 diabetes: a meta-analysis. *J Child Neurol* 26:1383–1391.

Bliss M. 1982. *The Discovery of Insulin*. Chicago, University of Chicago Press, pp. 109, 155, 157.

———. 1992. *Banting: A Biography*. 2nd ed. Toronto, University of Toronto Press, pp. 74–75.

Bolen S, Feldman L, Vassy J, Wilson L, Yeh H-C, Marinopoulos S, Wiley C, Selvin E, Wilson R, Bass EB, Brancati FL. 2007. Systematic review: comparative effectiveness and safety of oral medications for type 2 diabetes mellitus. *Ann Intern Med* 147:386–399.

Bolli G, De Feo P, Compagnucci P, Cartechini MG, Angeletti F, Santeusanio F, Brunetti P, Gerich JE. 1983. Abnormal glucose counterregulation in insulin dependent diabetes: interaction of anti-insulin antibodies and impaired glucagon and epinephrine secretion. *Diabetes* 32:134–141.

Bolli G, De Feo P, Perriello G, De Cosmo S, Ventura M, Campbell P, Brunetti P, Gerich JE. 1985. Role of hepatic autoregulation in defense against hypoglycemia in humans. *J Clin Invest* 75:162–1631.

Bolli GB, De Feo P, De Cosmo S, Perriello G, Ventura MM, Massi-Benedetti M, Santeusanio F, Gerich JE, Brunetti P. 1984. A reliable and reproducible test for adequate glucose counter-regulation in type 1 diabetes mellitus. *Diabetes* 33:732–737.

Bolli GB, Kerr D, Thomas R, Torlone E, Sola-Gazagnes A, Vitacolonna E, Selam JL, Home PD. 2009. Comparison of a multiple daily insulin injection regime (basal once-daily glargine plus mealtime lispro) and continuous subcutaneous insulin infusion (lispro) in type 1 diabetes. A randomized open parallel multicenter study. *Diabetes Care* 32:1170–1176.

Bonadonna RC, Heise T, Arbet-Engels C, Kapitza C, Avogaro A, Grimsby J, Zhi J, Grippo JF, Balena R. 2010. Piragliatin (R04389620), a novel glucokinase activator, lowers plasma glucose both in the postabsorptive state and after a glucose challenge in patients with type 2 diabetes mellitus: a mechanistic study. *J Clin Endocrinol Metab* 95:5028–5036.

Bonds DE, Miller ME, Bergenstal RM, Buse JB, Byington RP, Cutler JA, Dudl RJ, Ismail-Beigi F, Kimel AR, Hoogwerf B, Horowitz KR, Savage PJ, Seaquist ER, Simmons DL, Sivitz WI, Speril-Hillen JM, Sweeney ME. 2010. The association between symptomatic, severe hypoglycaemia and mortality in type 2 diabetes: retrospective epidemiological analysis of the ACCORD study. *BMJ* 340:b4909.

Bottini P, Boschetti E, Pampanelli S, Ciofetta M, Del Sindaco P, Scionti L, Brunetti P, Bolli GB. 1997. Contribution of autonomic neuropathy to reduced plasma adrenaline responses to hypoglycemia in IDDM. Evidence for a nonselective defect. *Diabetes* 46:814–823.

Boumezbeur F, Petersen KF, Cline GW, Mason GF, Behar KL, Shulman GI, Rothman DL. 2010. The contribution of blood lactate to brain energy metabolism in humans measured by dynamic ^{13}C nuclear magnetic resonance spectroscopy. *J Neurosci* 30:13983–13991.

Boyle JP, Thompson TJ, Gregg EW, Barker LE, Williamson DF. 2010. Projection of the year 2050 burden of diabetes in the US adult population: dynamic modeling of incidence, mortality and prediabetes prevalence. *Popul Health Metr* 8:29.

Boyle PJ, Cryer PE. 1991. Growth hormone, cortisol, or both are involved in defense against, but are not critical to recovery from, hypoglycemia. *Am J Physiol Endocrinol Metab* 260:E395–E402.

Boyle PJ, Justice K, Krentz AJ, Nagy RJ, Schade DS. 1993. Octreotide reverses hyperinsulinemia and prevents hypoglycemia induced by sulfonylurea overdoses. *J Clin Endocrinol Metab* 76:752–756.

Boyle PJ, Kempers SF, O'Connor AM, Nagy RJ. 1995. Brain glucose uptake and unawareness of hypoglycemia in patients with insulin dependent diabetes mellitus. *N Engl J Med* 333:1726–1731.

Boyle PJ, Nagy RJ, O'Connor AM, Kempers SF, Yeo RA, Qualls C. 1994. Adaptation in brain glucose uptake following recurrent hypoglycemia. *Proc Natl Acad Sci USA* 91:9352–9356.

Boyle PJ, Schwartz NS, Shah SD, Clutter WE, Cryer PE. 1988. Plasma glucose concentrations at the onset of hypoglycemic symptoms in patients with poorly controlled diabetes and in nondiabetics. *N Engl J Med* 318:1487–1492.

Boyle PJ, Shah SD, Cryer PE. 1989. Insulin, glucagon, and catecholamines in prevention of hypoglycemia during fasting in humans. *Am J Physiol Endocrinol Metab* 256:E651–E661.

Brambilla P, Bougneres PF, Santiago JV, Chaussain JL, Pouplard A, Castano L. 1987. Glucose counterregulation in pre-school-age diabetic children with recurrent hypoglycemia during conventional treatment. *Diabetes* 36:300–304.

Braun M, Ramracheya R, Amisten S, Bengtsson M, Moritoh Y, Zhang Q, Johnson PR, Rorsman P. 2009. Somatostatin release, electrical activity, membrane currents and exocytosis in human pancreatic delta cells. *Diabetologia* 52:1566–1578.

Breckenridge SM, Cooperberg BA, Arbeláez AM, Patterson BW, Cryer PE. 2007. Glucagon, in concert with insulin, supports the postabsorptive plasma glucose concentration in humans. *Diabetes* 56:2442–2448.

Bremer JP, Jauch-Chara K, Hallschmid M, Schmid S, Schultes B. 2009. Hypoglycemia unawareness in older compared with middle-aged patients with type 2 diabetes. *Diabetes Care* 32:1513–1517.

Briscoe VJ, Ertl AC, Tate DB, Blair HM, Davis SN. 2008a. Effects of the selective serotonin reuptake inhibitor, fluoxetine, on counterregulatory responses to hypoglycemia in individuals with T1DM. *Diabetes* 57:3315–3322.

Briscoe VJ, Ertl AC, Tate DB, Dawling S, Davis SN. 2008b. Effects of a selective serotonin reuptake inhibitor, fluoxetine, on counterregulatory responses to hypoglycemia in healthy individuals. *Diabetes* 57:2453–2460.

Brown AM, Sickmann HM, Fosgerau K, Lund TM, Schousboe A, Waagepetersen HS, Ransom BR. 2005. Astrocyte glycogen metabolism is required for neural activity during aglycemia or intense stimulation in mouse white matter. *J Neurosci Res* 79:74–80.

Bruce DG, Davis WA, Casey GP, Clarnette RM, Brown SGA, Jacobs IG, Almeida OP, Davis TME. 2009. Severe hypoglycaemia and cognitive impairment in older patients with diabetes: the Fremantle Diabetes Study. *Diabetologia* 52:1808–1815.

Bruce S, Tack C, Patel J, Pacak K, Goldstein DS. 2002. Local sympathetic function in human skeletal muscle and adipose tissue assessed by microdialysis. *Clin Auton Res* 12:13–19.

Budnitz DS, Lovegrove MC, Shehab N, Richards CL. 2011. Emergency hospitalizations for adverse drug events in older Americans. *N Engl J Med* 365:2002–2012.

Bulsara MK, Holman CDJ, van Bockxmeer FM, Davis EA, Gallego PH, Beilby JP, Palmer LJ, Choong C, Jones TW. 2007. The relationship between ACE genotype and risk of severe hypoglycaemia in a large population-based cohort of children and adolescents with type 1 diabetes. *Diabetologia* 50:965–971.

Burant CF, Viswanathan P, Marcinak J, Cao C, Vakilynejad M, Xie B, Leifke E. 2012. TAK-875 versus placebo or glimepiride in type 2 diabetes mellitus: a phase 2, randomised, double-blind, placebo-controlled trial. *Lancet* 379:1403–1411.

Caduff A, Lutz HU, Heinemann L, Di Benedetto G, Talary MS, Theander S. 2011. Dynamics of blood electrolytes in repeated hyper- and/or hypoglycaemic events in patients with type 1 diabetes. *Diabetologia* 54:2678–2689.

Campbell PJ, Bolli GB, Cryer PE, Gerich JE. 1985. Pathogenesis of the dawn phenomenon in patients with insulin-dependent diabetes mellitus. *N Engl J Med* 312:1473–1479.

Canada SE, Weaver SA, Sharpe SN, Pederson BA. 2011. Brain glycogen supercompensation in the mouse after recovery from insulin-induced hypoglycemia. *J Neurosci Res* 89:585–591.

Caprio S, Gerety G, Tamborlane WV, Jones T, Diamond M, Jacob R, Sherwin RS. 1991. Opiate blockade enhances hypoglycemic counterregulation in normal and insulin-dependent diabetic subjects. *Am J Physiol* 260:E852–E858.

Caprio S, Tamborlane WV, Zych K, Gerow K, Sherwin RS. 1993. Loss of potentiating effect of hypoglycemia on the glucagon response to hyperaminoacidemia in IDDM. *Diabetes* 42:550–555.

Castle JR, Engle JM, El Youssef J, Massoud RG, Yuen KCJ, Kagan R, Ward WK. 2010. Novel use of glucagon in a closed-loop system for prevention of hypoglycemia in type 1 diabetes. *Diabetes Care* 33:1282–1287.

Chelliah YR. 2000. Ventricular arrhythmias associated with hypoglycaemia. *Anaesth Intensive Care* 28:698–700.

Cherrington AD. 2001. Control of glucose production in vivo by insulin and glucagon. In *Handbook of Physiology*. Section 7, The Endocrine System. Volume II, The Endocrine Pancreas and Regulation of Metabolism. Jefferson LS, Cherrington AD, Eds. New York, Oxford University Press, pp. 759–785.

Chico A, Vidal-Rios P, Subirà M, Novials A. 2003. The continuous glucose monitoring system is useful for detecting unrecognized hypoglycemias in patients with type 1 and type 2 diabetes but is not better than frequent capillary glucose measurements for improving metabolic control. *Diabetes Care* 26:1153–1157.

Choi IY, Seaquist ER, Gruetter R. 2003. Effect of hypoglycemia on brain glycogen metabolism in vivo. *J Neurosci Res* 72:25–32.

Choudhary P, Geddes J, Freeman JV, Emery CJ, Heller SR, Frier BM. 2010. Frequency of biochemical hypoglycaemia in adults with type 1 diabetes with and without impaired awareness of hypoglycaemia: no identifiable difference using continuous glucose monitoring. *Diabet Med* 27:666–672.

Choudhary P, Lonnen K, Emergy CJ, MacDonald IA, MacLeod KM, Amiel SA, Heller SR. 2009. Comparing hormonal and symptomatic responses to experimental hypoglycaemia in insulin- and sulfonylurea-treated type 2 diabetes. *Diabet Med* 26:665–672.

Choudhary P, Shin J, Wang Y, Evans ML, Hammond PJ, Kerr D, Shaw JAM, Pickup JC, Amiel SA. 2011. Insulin pump therapy with automated insulin suspension in response to hypoglycemia. *Diabetes Care* 34:2023–2025.

Chow E, Heller SR. 2012. Pathophysiology of the effects of hypoglycemia on the cardiovascular system. *Diabetic Hypoglycemia* 5:3–8.

Christensen NJ, Norsk P. 2005. The fallacy of plasma nor-adrenaline spillover measurements. *Acta Physiol Scand* 183:333–334.

Clarke DD, Sokoloff L. 1994. Circulation and energy metabolism of the brain. In *Basic Neurochemistry: Molecular, Cellular and Medical Aspects,* 5th ed. Siegel G, Agranoff B, Albers RW, Molinoff P, Eds. New York, Raven Press, pp. 645–680.

Clarke WL, Cox DJ, Gonder-Frederick LA, Julian D, Schlundt D, Polonsky W. 1995. Reduced awareness of hypoglycemia in IDDM adults: a prospective study of hypoglycemia frequency and associated symptoms. *Diabetes Care* 18:517–522.

Clarke WL, Santiago JV, Thomas L, Ben-Galim E, Haymond MW, Cryer PE. 1979. Adrenergic mechanisms in recovery from hypoglycemia in man: adrenergic blockade. *Am J Physiol Endocrinol Metab* 236:E147–E152.

Colayco DC, Niu F, McCombs JS, Cheetham TC. 2011. A1C and cardiovascular outcomes in type 2 diabetes. A nested case-control study. *Diabetes Care* 34:77–83.

Cooke D, Hurel SJ, Casbard A, Steed L, Walker S, Meredith S, Nunn AJ, Manca A, Sculpher M, Barnard M, Kerr D, Weaver JU, Ahlquist J, Newman SP. 2009. Randomized controlled trial to assess the impact of continuous glucose monitoring on HbA(1c) in insulin-treated diabetes (MITRE Study). *Diabet Med* 26:540–547.

Cooperberg BA, Breckenridge SM, Arbeláez AM, Cryer PE. 2008. Terbutaline and the prevention of nocturnal hypoglycemia in type 1 diabetes. *Diabetes Care* 31:2271–2272.

Cooperberg BA, Cryer PE. 2009. β-cell-mediated signaling predominates over direct α-cell signaling in the regulation of glucagon secretion in humans. *Diabetes Care* 32:2275–2280.

————. 2010a. Insulin reciprocally regulates glucagon secretion in humans. *Diabetes* 59:2936–2940.

————. 2010b. Glucagon supports postabsorptive plasma glucose concentrations in humans with biologically optimal insulin levels. *Diabetes* 59:2941–2944.

Cox DJ, Fort D, Gonder-Frederick L, Clarke W, Mazze R, Weinger K, Ritterband L. 2009. Driving mishaps among individuals with type 1 diabetes. A prospective study. *Diabetes Care* 32:2177–2180.

Cox DJ, Gonder-Frederick L, Antoun B, Cryer PE, Clarke WL. 1993. Perceived symptoms in the recognition of hypoglycemia. *Diabetes Care* 16:519–527.

Cox DJ, Gonder-Frederick L, Ritterband L, Clarke W, Kovatchev BP. 2007. Prediction of severe hypoglycemia. *Diabetes Care* 30:1370–1373.

Cox DJ, Kovatchev B, Koev D, Koeva L, Dachev S, Tcharaktchiev D, Protopopova A, Gonder-Frederick L, Clarke W. 2004. Hypoglycemia anticipation, awareness and treatment training (HAATT) reduces occurrence of severe hypoglycemia among adults with type 1 diabetes mellitus. *Int J Behav Med* 11:212–218.

Cox DJ, Kovatchev BP, Anderson SM, Clarke WL, Gonder-Frederick LA. 2010. Type 1 diabetic drivers with and without a history of recurrent hypoglycemia-related driving mishaps. Physiological and performance differences during euglycemia and the induction of hypoglycemia. *Diabetes Care* 33:2430–2435.

Craft S, Newcomer J, Kanne S, Dagogo-Jack S, Cryer P, Sheline Y, Luby J, Dagogo-Jack A, Alderson A. 1996. Memory improvement following induced hyperinsulinemia in Alzheimer's disease. *Neurobiol Aging* 17:123–130.

Cranston I, Lomas J, Maran A, Macdonald I, Amiel SA. 1994. Restoration of hypoglycaemia awareness in patients with long-duration insulin-dependent diabetes. *Lancet* 344:283–287.

Cranston I, Reed LJ, Marsden PK, Amiel SA. 2001. Changes in regional brain ^{18}F-fluorodeoxyglucose uptake at hypoglycemia in type 1 diabetic men associated with hypoglycemia unawareness and counter-regulatory failure. *Diabetes* 50:2329–2336.

Cryer PE. 1981. Glucose counterregulation in man. *Diabetes* 30:261–264.

———. 1992. Iatrogenic hypoglycemia as a cause of hypoglycemia-associated autonomic failure in IDDM: a vicious cycle. *Diabetes* 41:255–260.

———. 1993. Catecholamines, pheochromocytoma and diabetes. *Diabetes Reviews* 1:309–317.

———. 1997. *Hypoglycemia: Pathophysiology, Diagnosis and Treatment.* New York, Oxford University Press, pp. 1–177.

———. 2001. The prevention and correction of hypoglycemia. In *Handbook of Physiology.* Section 7, The Endocrine System. Volume II, The Endocrine Pancreas and Regulation of Metabolism. Jefferson LS, Cherrington AD, Eds. New York, Oxford University Press, pp. 1057–1092.

———. 2004. Diverse causes of hypoglycemia-associated autonomic failure in diabetes. *N Engl J Med* 350:2272–2279.

———. 2005. Mechanisms of hypoglycemia-associated autonomic failure and its component syndromes in diabetes. *Diabetes* 54:3592–3601.

———. 2006a. Hypoglycaemia: the limiting factor in the glycaemic management of the critically ill? *Diabetologia* 49:1722–1725.

———. 2006b. Mechanisms of sympathoadrenal failure and hypoglycemia in diabetes. *J Clin Invest* 116:1470–1473.

———. 2007. Hypoglycemia, functional brain failure, and brain death. *J Clin Invest* 117:868–870.

———. 2008. The barrier of hypoglycemia in diabetes. *Diabetes* 57:3169–3176.

———. 2009. Preventing hypoglycaemia: what is the appropriate glucose alert value? *Diabetologia* 52:35–37.

———. 2010. Hypoglycemia in diabetes. In Textbook of Diabetes, 4th Edition. Holt RIG, Cockram C, Flyvbjerg A, Goldstein BJ, Eds. Oxford, UK, Wiley-Blackwell, pp. 528–545.

———. 2011a. Hypoglycemia. In *Williams Textbook of Endocrinology*. 12th ed. Melmed S, Polonsky S, Larsen PR, Kronenberg H, Eds. Philadelphia, Elsevier, pp. 1552–1577.

———. 2011b. Elimination of hypoglycemia from the lives of people with diabetes. *Diabetes* 60:24–27.

———. 2011c. Death during intensive glycemic therapy of diabetes: mechanisms and implications. *Am J Med* 124:993–996.

———. 2012. Glucagon in the pathogenesis of hypoglycemia and hyperglycemia in diabetes. *Endocrinology* 153:1039–1048.

Cryer PE, Axelrod L, Grossman AB, Heller SR, Montori VM, Seaquist ER, Service FJ. 2009. Evaluation and management of adult hypoglycemic disorders. *J Clin Endocrinol Metab* 94:709–728.

Cryer PE, Davis SN, Shamoon H. 2003. Hypoglycemia in diabetes. *Diabetes Care* 26:1902–1912.

Cummins E, Royle P, Snaith A, Greene A, Robertson L, McIntyre L, Waugh N. 2010. Clinical effectiveness and cost-effectiveness of continuous subcutaneous insulin infusion for diabetes: systematic review and economic evaluation. *Health Technol Assess* 14:iii–iv, xi–xvi, 1–181.

Currie CJ, Peters JR, Tynan A, Evans M, Heine RJ, Bracco OL, Zagar T, Poole CD. 2010. Survival as a function of HbA1C in people with type 2 diabetes: a retrospective cohort study. *Lancet* 375:481–489.

Dagogo-Jack S, Rattarasarn C, Cryer PE. 1994. Reversal of hypoglycemia unawareness, but not defective glucose counterregulation, in IDDM. *Diabetes* 43:1426–1434.

Dagogo-Jack SE, Craft S, Cryer PE. 1993. Hypoglycemia-associated autonomic failure in insulin-dependent diabetes mellitus. *J Clin Invest* 91:819–828.

Dalsgaard MK. 2006. Fuelling cerebral activity in exercising man. *J Cerebral Blood Flow Metab* 26:731–750.

Danne T, Kordonouri O, Holder M, Haberland H, Golembowski S, Remus K, Bläsig S, Wadien T, Zierow S, Hartmann R, Thomas A. 2011. Prevention of hypoglycemia by using low glucose suspend function in sensor-augmented pump therapy. *Diabetes Technol Ther* 13:1129–1134.

Davis SN, Mann S, Briscoe VJ, Ertl AC, Tate DB. 2009. Effects of intensive therapy and antecedent hypoglycemia on counterregulatory responses to hypoglycemia in type 2 diabetes. *Diabetes* 58:701–709.

Davis SN, Shavers C, Costa F, Mosqueda-Garcia R. 1996. Role of cortisol in the pathogenesis of deficient counterregulation after antecedent hypoglycemia in normal humans. *J Clin Invest* 98:680–691.

Davis SN, Shavers C, Davis B, Costa F. 1997a. Prevention of an increase in plasma cortisol during hypoglycemia preserves subsequent counterregulatory responses. *J Clin Invest* 100:429–438.

Davis SN, Shavers C, Mosqueda-Garcia R, Costa F. 1997b. Effects of differing antecedent hypoglycemia on subsequent counterregulation in normal humans. *Diabetes* 46:1328–1335.

Davis WA, Brown SGA, Jacobs IG, Bulsara M, Beilby J, Bruce DG, Davis TME. 2011. Angiotensin converting enzyme insertion/deletion polymorphism and severe hypoglycemia complicating type 2 diabetes: the Fremantle Diabetes Study. *J Clin Endocrinol Metab* 96:E696–E700.

De Feo P, Perriello G, De Cosmo S, Ventura MM, Campbell PJ, Brunetti P, Gerich JE, Bolli GB. 1986. Comparison of glucose counterregulation during short-term and prolonged hypoglycemia in normal humans. *Diabetes* 35:563–569.

De Feo P, Perriello G, Torlone E, Fanelli C, Ventura MM, Santeusanio F, Brunetti P, Gerich JE, Bolli GB. 1991a. Evidence against important catecholamine compensation for absent glucagon counterregulation. *Am J Physiol Endocrinol Metab* 260:E203–E212.

———. 1991b. Contribution of adrenergic mechanisms to glucose counterregulation in humans. *Am J Physiol Endocrinol Metab* 261:E725–E736.

De Feo P, Perriello G, Torlone E, Ventura MM, Fanelli C, Santeusanio F, Brunetti P, Gerich JE, Bolli GB. 1989b. Contribution of cortisol to glucose counterregulation in humans. *Am J Physiol Endocrinol Metab* 257:E35–E42.

De Feo P, Perriello G, Torlone E, Ventura MM, Santeusanio F, Brunetti P, Gerich JE, Bolli GB. 1989a. Demonstration of a role for growth hormone in glucose counterregulation. *Am J Physiol Endocrinol Metab* 256:E835–E843.

De Feyter HM, Shulman GI, Rothman DL, Petersen KF. 2012. Increased brain uptake of lactate in type 1 diabetic patients with hypoglycemia unawareness (abstract). *Diabetes* 61:A33.

DeFronzo RA. 2011. Bromocriptine: a sympatholytic, D2-dopamine agonist for the treatment of type 2 diabetes. *Diabetes Care* 34:789–794. (Erratum in: *Diabetes Care* 2011. 34:1442. Dosage error in article text.)

de Galan BE, De Mol P, Wennekes L, Schouwenberg BJJ, Smits P. 2006. Preserved sensitivity to β₂-adrenergic receptor agonists in patients with type 1 diabetes mellitus and hypoglycemia unawareness. *J Clin Endocrinol Metab* 91:2878–2881.

de Galan BE, Rietjens SJ, Tack CJ, Van der Werf SP, Sweep CGJ, Lenders JWM, Smits P. 2003. Antecedent adrenaline attenuates the responsiveness to, but not the release of, counterregulatory hormones during subsequent hypoglycemia. *J Clin Endocrinol Metab* 88:5462–5467.

de Galan BE, Tack CJ, Willemsen JJ, Sweep CGJ, Smits P, Lenders JWM. 2004. Plasma metanephrine levels are decreased in type 1 diabetic patients with a severely impaired epinephrine response to hypoglycemia, indicating reduced stores of epinephrine. *J Clin Endocrinol Metab* 89:2057–2061.

de Heer J, Holst JJ. 2007. Sulfonylurea compounds uncouple the glucose dependence of the insulinotropic effect of glucagon-like peptide1. *Diabetes* 56:438–443.

de Vries MG, Arseneau LM, Lawson ME, Beverly JL. 2003. Extracellular glucose in rat ventromedial hypothalamus during acute and recurrent hypoglycemia. *Diabetes* 52:2767–2773.

Deary IJ, Hepburn DA, MacLeod KM, Frier BM. 1993. Partitioning of the symptoms of hypoglycaemia using multi-sample confirmatory factor analysis. *Diabetologia* 36:771–777.

Deckert T, Poulsen JE, Larsen M. 1978. Prognosis of diabetics with diabetes before the age of 31. I. Survival, cause of deaths and complications. *Diabetologia* 14:363–370.

DeRosa MA, Cryer PE. 2004. Hypoglycemia and the sympathoadrenal system: neurogenic symptoms are largely the result of sympathetic neural, rather than adrenomedullary, activation. *Am J Physiol Endocrinol Metab* 287:E32–E41.

Diabetes Control and Complications Trial Research Group [DCCT]. 1986. The Diabetes Control and Complications Trial: design and methodologic considerations for the feasibility phase. *Diabetes* 35:530–545.

———. 1991. Epidemiology of severe hypoglycemia in the Diabetes Control and Complications Trial. *Am J Med* 90:450–459.

———. 1993. The effect of intensive treatment of diabetes on the development and progression of long-term complications in insulin dependent diabetes mellitus. *N Engl J Med* 329:977–986.

————. 1995. The relationship of glycemic exposure (HbA$_{1C}$) to the risk of development and progression of retinopathy in the Diabetes Control and Complications Trial. *Diabetes* 44:968–983.

————. 1996. Influence of intensive diabetes treatment on quality-of-life outcomes in the Diabetes Control and Complications Trial. *Diabetes Care* 19:195–203.

————. 1997. Hypoglycemia in the Diabetes Control and Complications Trial. *Diabetes* 46:271–286.

Diabetes Control and Complications Trial/Epidemiology of Diabetes Interventions and Complications (DCCT/EDIC) Research Group. 2000. Retinopathy and nephropathy in patients with type 1 diabetes four years after a trial of intensive therapy. *N Engl J Med* 342:381-389.

————. 2005. Intensive diabetes treatment and cardiovascular disease in patients with type 1 diabetes. *N Engl J Med* 353:2643-2653.

————. 2007. Long-term effect of diabetes and its treatment on cognitive function. *N Engl J Med* 356:1842-1852.

Diabetes Research in Children Network (DirecNet) Study Group. 2003. A multicenter study of the accuracy of the One Touch Ultra home glucose meter in children with type 1 diabetes. *Diabetes Technol Ther* 5:933-941.

Diem P, Redmon JB, Abid M, Moran A, Sutherland DER, Halter JB, Robertson RP. 1990. Glucagon, catecholamine and pancreatic polypeptide secretion in type 1 diabetic recipients of pancreatic allografts. *J Clin Invest* 86:2008-2013.

Donnelly LA, Morris AD, Frier BM, Ellis JD, Donnan PT, Durrant R, Band MM, Reekie G, Leese GP, for the DARTS/MEMO Collaboration. 2005. Frequency and predictors of hypoglycaemia in type 1 and insulin-treated type 2 diabetes: a population-based study. *Diabet Med* 22:749-755.

Dougherty PP, Klein-Schwartz W. 2010. Octreotide's role in the management of sulfonylurea-induced hypoglycemia. *J Med Toxicol* 6:199-206.

Duckworth W, Abraira C, Moritz T, Reda D, Emanuele N, Reaven PD, et al. for the Veterans Affairs Diabetes Therapy [VADT] Investigators. 2009. Glucose control and vascular complications in veterans with type 2 diabetes. *N Engl J Med* 360:129-139.

Dunn JT, Cranston I, Marsden PK, Amiel SA, Reed LJ. 2007. Attenuation of amygdala and frontal cortical responses to low blood glucose concentration in asymptomatic hypoglycemia in type 1 diabetes. *Diabetes* 56:2766-2773.

Eaton RP, Allen RC, Schade DS, Erickson KM, Standefer J. 1980. Prehepatic insulin production in man: kinetic analysis using peripheral connecting peptide behavior. *J Clin Endocrinol Metab* 51:520-528.

Edgerton DS, Cherrington AD. 2011. Glucagon as a critical factor in the pathology of diabetes. *Diabetes* 60:377-380.

Edgerton DS, Lautz M, Scott M, Everett CA, Stettler KM, Neal DW, Chu CA, Cherrington AD. 2006. Insulin's direct effects on the liver dominate the control of hepatic glucose production. *J Clin Invest* 116:521-527.

Eeg-Olofsson K, Cederholm J, Nilsson PM, Zethelius B, Svensson A-M, Gudbjörnsdóttir S, Eliasson B. 2010. New aspects of HbA$_{1C}$ as a risk factor for cardiovascular diseases in type 2 diabetes: an observational study from the Swedish National Diabetes Register (NDR). *J Intern Med* 268:471–482.

Egger M, Davey Smith G, Stettler C, Diem P. 1997. Risk of adverse effects of intensified treatment in insulin-dependent diabetes mellitus: a meta-analysis. *Diabet Med* 14:919–928.

Eisenhofer G. 2005. Sympathetic nerve function: assessment of radioisotope dilution analysis. *Clin Auton Res* 15:264–283.

Eisenhofer G, Kopin IJ, Goldstein DS. 2004. Catecholamine metabolism: a contemporary view with implications for physiology and medicine. *Pharmacological Reviews* 56:331–349.

El-Khatib FH, Russell SJ, Nathan DM, Sutherlin RG, Damiano ER. 2010. A bihormonal closed-loop artificial pancreas for type 1 diabetes. *Sci Transl Med* 2:27ra27.

Ertl AC, Davis SN. 2004. Evidence for a vicious cycle of exercise and hypoglycemia in type 1 diabetes mellitus. *Diabetes Metab Res Rev* 20:124–130.

Evers IM, ter Braak EWMT, de Valk HW, van der Schoot B, Janssen N, Visser GHA. 2002. Risk indicators predictive of severe hypoglycemia during the first trimester of type 1 diabetic pregnancy. *Diabetes Care* 25:554–559.

Fagius J. 2003. Sympathetic nerve activity in metabolic control: some basic concepts. *Acta Physiol Scand* 177:337–343.

Falconnier Bendik C, Keller U, Moriconi N, Gessler A, Schindler Ch, Zulewski H, Ruiz J, Puder JJ. 2009. Training in flexible intensive insulin therapy improves quality of life, decreases the risk of hypoglycaemia and ameliorates poor metabolic control in patients with type 1 diabetes. *Diabetes Res Clin Pract* 83:327–333.

Fanelli C, Pampanelli S, Epifano L, Rambotti AM, Ciofetta M, Modarelli F, Di Vincenzo A, Annibale B, Lepore M, Lalli C, Del Sindaco P, Brunetti P, Bolli GB. 1994a. Relative roles of insulin and hypoglycaemia on induction of neuroendocrine responses to, symptoms of, and deterioration of cognitive function in hypoglycaemia in male and female humans. *Diabetologia* 37:797–807.

Fanelli C, Pampanelli S, Epifano L, Rambotti AM, Di Vincenzo A, Modarelli F, Ciofetta M, Lepore M, Annibale B, Torlone E, Perriello G, De Feo P, Santeusanio F, Brunetti P, Bolli GB. 1994b. Long-term recovery from unawareness, deficient counterregulation and lack of cognitive dysfunction during hypoglycemia, following institution of rational, intensive therapy in IDDM. *Diabetologia* 37:1265–1276.

Fanelli CG, De Feo P, Porcellati F, Perriello G, Torlone E, Santeusanio F, Brunetti P, Bolli GB. 1992. Adrenergic mechanisms contribute to the late phase of hypoglycemic glucose counterregulation in humans by stimulating lipolysis. *J Clin Invest* 89:2005–2013.

Fanelli CG, Dence CS, Markham J, Videen TO, Paramore DS, Cryer PE, Powers WJ. 1998. Blood-to-brain glucose transport and cerebral glucose metabolism are not reduced in poorly controlled type 1 diabetes. *Diabetes* 47:1444–1450.

Fanelli CG, Epifano L, Rambotti AM, Pampanelli S, Di Vincenzo A, Modarelli F, Lepore M, Annibale B, Ciofetta M, Bottini P, Porcellati F, Scionti L, Santeusanio F, Brunetti P, Bolli GB. 1993. Meticulous prevention of hypoglycemia normalizes the glycemic thresholds and magnitude of most of neuroendocrine responses to, symptoms of, and cognitive function during hypoglycemia in intensively treated patients with short-term IDDM. *Diabetes* 42:1683–1689.

Fanelli CG, Paramore DS, Hershey T, Terkamp C, Ovalle F, Craft S, Cryer PE. 1998. Impact of nocturnal hypoglycemia on hypoglycemic cognitive dysfunction in type 1 diabetes. Diabetes 47:1920–1927.

Fatourechi MM, Kudva YC, Murad MH, Elamin MB, Tabini CC, Montori VM. 2009. Hypoglycemia with intensive insulin therapy. A systematic review and meta-analysis of randomized trials of continuous subcutaneous insulin infusion versus multiple daily injections. *J Clin Endocrinol* Metab 94:729–740.

Feltbower RG, Bodansky HJ, Patterson CC, Parslow RC, Stephenson CR, Reynolds C, McKinney PA. 2008. Acute complications and drug misuse are important causes of death for children and young adults with type 1 diabetes. *Diabetes Care* 31:922–926.

Ferner RE, Neil HA. 1988. Sulfonylureas and hypoglycemia. *BMJ* 296:949–950.

Ferrannini E. 2012. Physiology of glucose homeostasis and insulin therapy in type 1 and type 2 diabetes. *Endocrinol Metab Clin N Am* 41:25–39.

Ferrannini E, Ramos SJ, Salsali A, Tang W, List JF. 2010. Dapagliflozin monotherapy in type 2 diabetic patients with inadequate glycemic control by diet and exercise. A randomized, double-blind, placebo-controlled, phase 3 trial. *Diabetes Care* 33:2217–2224.

Freathy RM, Lonnen KF, Steele AM, Minton JAL, Frayling TM, Hattersley AT, MacLeod KM. 2006. The impact of the angiotensin-converting enzyme insertion/deletion polymorphism on severe hypoglycemia in type 2 diabetes. *Rev Diabet Stud* 3:76–81.

Frier BM, Fisher BM. 1999. Impaired hypoglycemia awareness. In *Hypoglycaemia in Clinical Diabetes*. Fisher BM, Frier BM, Eds. Chichester, UK, John Wiley & Sons, pp. 111–146.

Frier BM, Schernthaner G, Heller SR. 2011. Hypoglycemia and cardiovascular risks. Diabetes Care 34(Suppl 2):S132-S137.

Fritsche A, Stefan N, Häring H, Gerich J, Stumvoll M. 2001. Avoidance of hypoglycemia restores hypoglycemia awareness by increasing β-adrenergic sensitivity in type 1 diabetes. *Ann Intern Med* 134:729–736.

Fukuda M, Tanaka A, Tahara Y, Ikegami H, Yamamoto Y, Kumahara Y, Shima K. 1988. Correlation between minimal secretory capacity of pancreatic β-cells and stability of diabetic control. *Diabetes* 37:81–88.

Gaede P, Vedel P, Larsen N, Jensen GVH, Parving H-H, Pedersen O. 2003. Multifactorial intervention and cardiovascular disease in patients with type 2 diabetes. *N Engl J Med* 348:383–393.

Galassetti P, Mann S, Tate D, Neill RA, Costa F, Wasserman DH, Davis SN. 2001. Effects of antecedent prolonged exercise on subsequent counterregulatory responses to hypoglycemia. *Am J Physiol Endocrinol Metab* 280:E908–E917.

Gangji AS, Cukierman T, Gerstein HC, Goldsmith GH, Clase CM. 2007. A systematic review and meta-analysis of hypoglycemia and cardiovascular events. *Diabetes Care* 30:389–394.

Garber AJ, Cryer PE, Santiago JV, Haymond MW, Pagliara AS, Kipnis DM. 1976. The role of adrenergic mechanisms in the substrate and hormonal response to insulin-induced hypoglycemia in man. *J Clin Invest* 58:7–15.

Garber AJ, King AB, Del Prato S, Sreenan S, Balci MK, Muñoz-Torres M, Rosenstock J, Endahl LA, Francisco AMO, Hollander P, on behalf of the NN1250-3582 (BEGIN BB T2D) Trial Investigators. 2012. Insulin degludec, an ultra-longacting basal insulin, versus insulin glargine in basal-bolus treatment with mealtime insulin aspart in type 2 diabetes (BEGIN Basal-Bolus Type 2): a phase 3, randomised, open-label, treat-to-target non-inferiority trial. *Lancet* 379:1498–1507.

Garg S, Brazg RL, Bailey TS, Buckingham BA, Slover RH, Klonoff DC, Shin J, Welsh JB, Kaufman FR. 2012. Reduction in duration of hypoglycemia by automatic suspension of insulin delivery: the in-clinic ASPIRE study. *Diabetes Technol Ther* 14:205–209.

Gaziano JM, Cincotta AH, O'Connor CM, Ezrokhi M, Rutty D, Ma ZJ, Scranton RE. 2010. Randomized clinical trial of quick-release bromocriptine among patients with type 2 diabetes on overall safety and cardiovascular outcomes. *Diabetes Care.* 33:1503–1508.

Geddes J, Schopman JE, Zammitt NN, Frier BM. 2008. Prevalence of impaired awareness of hypoglycaemia in adults with type 1 diabetes. *Diabet Med* 25:501–504.

Gerich J, Davis J, Lorenzi M, Rizza R, Bohannon N, Karam J, Lewis S, Kaplan R, Schultz T, Cryer P. 1979. Hormonal mechanisms of recovery from insulin-induced hypoglycemia in man. *Am J Physiol Endocrinol Metab* 236:E380–E385.

Gerich JE. 1988. Glucose counterregulation and its impact on diabetes mellitus. *Diabetes* 37:1608–1617.

———. 1989. Oral hypoglycemic agents. *N Engl J Med* 321:1231–1245.

———. 2010. Role of the kidney in normal glucose homeostasis and in the hyperglycaemia of diabetes mellitus: therapeutic implications. *Diabet Med* 27:136–142.

Gerich JE, Charles MA, Grodsky GM. 1974. Characterization of the effects of arginine and glucose on glucagon and insulin release from the perfused rat pancreas. *J Clin Invest* 54:833–841.

Gerich JE, Langlois M, Noacco C, Karam J, Forsham P. 1973. Lack of glucagon response to hypoglycemia in diabetes: evidence for an intrinsic pancreatic alpha-cell defect. *Science* 182:171–173.

Gerich JE, Meyer C, Woerle HJ, Stumvoll M. 2001. Renal gluconeogenesis. *Diabetes Care* 24:382–391.

Gill GV, Woodward A, Casson IF, Weston PJ. 2009. Cardiac arrhythmia and nocturnal hypoglycaemia in type 1 diabetes— the 'dead in bed' syndrome revisited. *Diabetologia* 52:42–45.

Giménez M, Gilabert R, Monteagudo J, Alonso A, Casamitjana R, Paré C, Conget I. 2011. Repeated episodes of hypoglycemia as a potential aggravating factor for pre-clinical atherosclerosis in subjects with type 1 diabetes. *Diabetes Care* 34:198–203.

Giménez M, Lara M, Jiménez A, Conget I. 2009. Glycemic profile characteristics and frequency of impaired awareness of hypoglycaemia in subjects with T1D and repeated hypoglycaemic events. *Acta Diabetol* 46:291–293.

Gjessing HJ, Matzen LE, Faber OK, Frølund A. 1989. Fasting plasma C-peptide, glucagon stimulated plasma C-peptide and urinary C-peptide in relation to clinical type of diabetes. *Diabetologia* 32:305–311.

Gold AE, MacLeod KM, Frier BM. 1994. Frequency of severe hypoglycemia in patients with type 1 diabetes and impaired awareness of hypoglycemia. *Diabetes Care* 17:697–703.

Goldberg PA, Weiss R, McCrimmon RJ, Hintz EV, Dziura J, Sherwin RS. 2006. Antecedent hypercortisolemia is not primarily responsible for generating hypoglycemia-associated autonomic failure. *Diabetes* 55:1121–1126.

Goldman D. 1940. The electrocardiogram in insulin shock. *Arch Int Med* 66:93–108.

Goldstein DS, Kopin IJ. 2008. Adrenomedullary, adrenocortical, and sympathoneural responses to stressors: a meta-analysis. *Endocr Regul* 42:111–119.

Gonder-Frederick LA, Fisher CD, Ritterband LM, Cox DJ, Hou L, DasGupta AA, Clarke WL. 2006. Predictors of fear of hypoglycemia in adolescents with type 1 diabetes and their parents. *Pediatr Diabetes* 7:215–222.

Gosmanov NR, Szoke E, Israelian Z, Smith T, Cryer PE, Gerich JE, Meyer C. 2005. Role of the decrement in intraislet insulin for the glucagon response to hypoglycemia in humans. *Diabetes Care* 28:1124–1131.

Gough SCL. 2007. A review of human and analogue insulin trials. *Diabetes Res Clin Pract* 77:1–15.

Graveling AJ, Frier BM. 2009. Hypoglycaemia: an overview. *Primary Care Diabetes.* 3:131–139.

Grissom N, Bhatnagar S. 2009. Habituation to repeated stress: get used to it. *Neurobiol Learning Memory* 92:215–224.

Gromada J, Franklin I, Wollheim CB. 2007. Alpha cells of the endocrine pancreas: 35 years of research, but the enigma remains. *Endocrine Reviews* 28:84–116.

Gruetter R. 2003. Glycogen: the forgotten cerebral energy store. *J Neurosci Res* 74:179–183.

Guillod L, Comte-Perret S, Monbaron D, Gaillard RC, Ruiz J. 2007. Nocturnal hypoglycaemias in type 1 diabetic patients: what can we learn with continuous glucose monitoring? *Diabetes Metab* 33:360–365.

Gunning RR, Garber AJ. 1978. Bioactivity of instant glucose. Failure of absorption through oral mucosa. *JAMA* 240:1611–1612.

Gürlek A, Erbas T, Gedik O. 1999. Frequency of severe hypoglycaemia in type 1 and type 2 diabetes during conventional insulin therapy. *Exp Clin Endocrinol Diabetes* 107:220–224.

Gustavson SM, Chu SA, Nishizawa M, Farmer B, Neal D, Yang Y, Vaughan S, Donahue EP, Flakoll P, Cherrington AD. 2003. Glucagon's actions are modified by the combination of epinephrine and gluconeogenic precursor infusion. *Am J Physiol Endocrinol Metab* 285:E534–E544.

Hauge-Evans AC, King AJ, Carmignac D, Richardson CC, Robinson ICAF, Low MJ, Christie MR, Persaud SJ, Jones PM. 2009. Somatostatin secreted by islet δ-cells fulfills multiple roles as a paracrine regulator of islet function. *Diabetes* 58:403–411.

Havlin CE, Cryer PE. 1987. Nocturnal hypoglycemia does not result commonly in major morning hyperglycemia in patients with diabetes mellitus. *Diabetes Care* 10:141–147.

Haymond MW, Schreiner B. 2001. Mini-dose glucagon rescue to children with type 1 diabetes. *Diabetes Care* 24:643–645.

Heller S, Buse J, Fisher M, Garg S, Marre M, Merker L, Renard E, Russell-Jones D, Philotheou A, Francisco AMO, Pei H, Bode B, on behalf of the BEGIN Basal-Bolus Type 1 Trial Investigators. 2012. Insulin degludec, an ultra-longacting basal insulin, versus insulin glargine in basal-bolus treatment with mealtime insulin aspart in type 1 diabetes (Begin Basal-Bolus Type 1): A phase 3, randomised, open-label, treat-to-target non-inferiority trial. *Lancet* 379:1489–1497.

Heller S, Damm P, Mersebach H, Skjøth TV, Kaaja R, Hod M, Durán-Garcia, McCance D, Mathiesen ER. 2010. Hypoglycemia in type 1 diabetic pregnancy. *Diabetes Care* 33:473–477.

Heller SR, Cryer PE. 1991a. Hypoinsulinemia is not critical to glucose recovery from hypoglycemia in humans. *Am J Physiol Endocrinol Metab* 261:E41–E48.

———. 1991b. Reduced neuroendocrine and symptomatic responses to subsequent hypoglycemia after one episode of hypoglycemia in nondiabetic humans. *Diabetes* 40:223–226.

Hemmingsen B, Lund SS, Gluud C, Vaag A, Almdal T, Hemmingsen C, Wetterslev J. 2011. Targeting intensive glycaemic control versus targeting conventional glycaemic control for type 2 diabetes mellitus. *Cochrane Database of Systemic Reviews* Issue 6, Art. No. CD008143. doi: 10.1002/14651858. CD008143. pub 2.

Henderson JN, Allen KV, Deary IJ, Frier BM. 2003. Hypoglycaemia in insulin-treated type 2 diabetes: frequency, symptoms and impaired awareness. *Diabet Med* 20:1016–1021.

Hepburn DA, MacLeod KM, Pell AC, Scougal IJ, Frier BM. 1993. Frequency and symptoms of hypoglycaemia experienced by patients with type 2 diabetes treated with insulin. *Diabet Med* 10:231–237.

Hermanides J, De Vries JH. 2010. Sense and nonsense in sensors. *Diabetologia* 53:593–596.

Hermanides J, Phillip M, DeVries JH. 2011. Current application of continuous glucose monitoring in the treatment of diabetes. Pros and cons. *Diabetes Care* 34(Suppl 2):S197–S201.

Hershey T, Perantie DC, Warren SL, Zimmerman EC, Sadler M, White NH. 2005. Frequency and timing of severe hypoglycemia affects spatial memory in children with type 1 diabetes. *Diabetes Care* 28:2372–2377.

Hershey T, Perantie DC, Wu J, Weaver PM, Black KJ, White NH. 2010. Hippocampal volumes in youth with type 1 diabetes. *Diabetes* 59:236–241.

Herzog RI, Chan O, Yu S, Dziura J, McNay EC, Sherwin RS. 2008. Effect of acute and recurrent hypoglycemia on changes in brain glycogen concentration. *Endocrinology* 149:1499–1504.

Herzog RI, Jiang L, Mason G, Behar K, Rothman D, Sherwin RS. 2009. Increased brain lactate utilization following exposure to recurrent hypoglycemia (abstract). *Diabetes* 58:A14.

Herzog RI, Sherwin RS, Rothman DL. 2011. Insulin-induced hypoglycemia and its effect on the brain. Unraveling metabolism by in vivo nuclear magnetic resonance. *Diabetes* 60:1856–1858.

Hirsch IB. 2005. Insulin analogues. *N Engl J Med* 352:174–183.

Hirsch IB, Marker JC, Smith L, Spina RJ, Parvin CA, Holloszy JO, Cryer PE. 1991. Insulin and glucagon in the prevention of hypoglycemia during exercise in humans. *Am J Physiol Endocrinol Metab* 260:E695–E704.

Hirsch IB, Smith LJ, Havlin CE, Shah SD, Clutter WE, Cryer PE. 1990. Failure of nocturnal hypoglycemia to cause daytime hyperglycemia in patients with IDDM. *Diabetes Care* 13:133–142.

Hoffman RP, Singer-Granick C, Drash AL, Becker DJ. 1994. Abnormal alpha cell hypoglycemic recognition in children with insulin dependent diabetes mellitus (IDDM). *J Pediatr Endocrinol* 7:225–234.

Høi-Hansen T, Pedersen-Bjergaard U, Andersen RD, Kristensen PL, Thomsen C, Kjær T, Høgenhaven H, Smed A, Holst JJ, Dela F, Boomsma F, Thorsteinsson B. 2009. Cognitive performance, symptoms and counter-regulation during hypoglycaemia in patients with type 1 diabetes and high or low renin-angiotensin system activity. *J Renin Angiotensin Aldosterone Syst* 10:216–229.

Høi-Hansen T, Pedersen-Bjergaard U, Thorsteinsson B. 2010. Classification of hypoglycemia awareness in people with type 1 diabetes in clinical practice. *J Diabetes Complications* 24:392–397.

Holman RR, Farmer AJ, Davies MJ, Levy JC, Darbyshire JL, Keenan JF, Paul SK, for the 4T Study Group. 2009. Three-year efficacy of complex insulin regimens in type 2 diabetes. *N Engl J Med* 361:1736–1747.

Holman RR, Paul SK, Ethel MA, Matthews DR, Neil HAW. 2008. 10-year follow-up of intensive glucose control in type 2 diabetes. *N Engl J Med* 359:1577–1589.

Holst JJ. 2007. The physiology of glucagon-like peptide 1. Physiol Rev 87:1409–1439.

Holstein A, Egberts EH. 2003. Risk of hypoglycaemia with oral antidiabetic agents in patients with type 2 diabetes. *Exp Clin Endocrinol Metab* 111:405–414.

Holstein A, Patzer OM, Machalke K, Holstein JD, Stumvoll M, Kovacs P. 2012. Substantial increase in incidence of severe hypoglycemia between 1997-2000 and 2007-2010. *Diabetes Care* 35:972–975.

Holstein A, Plaschke A, Böttcher Y, Stumvoll M, Kovacs P. 2006. The insertion/deletion polymorphism in the angio-tensin-converting enzyme gene and hypoglycemia aware-ness in patients with type 1 diabetes. *Horm Metab Res* 38:603–606.

Holstein A, Plaschke A, Egberts E-H. 2003. Clinical charac-terization of severe hypoglycaemia: a prospective popula-tion-based study. *Exp Clin Endocrinol Diabetes* 111:364–369.

Horvath K, Jeitler K, Berghold A, Ebrahim SH, Gratzer TW, Plank J, Kaiser T, Pieber TR, Siebenhofer A. 2007. Long-acting insulin analogues versus NPH insulin (human iso-phane insulin) for type 2 diabetes. Cochrane Database of

Systematic Reviews. Issue 2. Art. No. CD005613. doi: 10.1002/14651858.CD005613.pub3.

Hovorka R, Allen JM, Elleri D, Chassin LJ, Harris J, Xing D, Kollman C, Hovorka T, Larsen AMF, Nodale M, De Palma A, Wilinska ME, Acerini CL, Dunger DB. 2010. Manual closed-loop insulin delivery in children and adolescents with type 1 diabetes: a phase 2 randomized crossover trial. *Lancet* 375:743–751.

Hovorka R, Kumareswaran K, Harris J, Allen JM, Elleri D, Xing D, Kollman C, Nodale M, Murphy HR, Dunger DB, Amiel SA, Heller SR, Wilinska ME, Evans ML. 2011. Overnight closed loop insulin delivery (artificial pancreas) in adults with type 1 diabetes: crossover randomised controlled studies. *BMJ* 342:d1855. doi: 10.1136/bmj.d1855

Huang ES, Liu JY, Moffet HN, John PM, Karter AJ. 2011. Glycemic control, complications, and death in older diabetic patients. *Diabetes Care* 34:1329–1336.

Hyder F, Patel AB, Gjedde A, Rothman DL, Behar KL, Shulman RG. 2006. Neuronal-glial glucose oxidation and glutaminergic-GABAergic function. *J Cerebr Blood Flow Metab* 26:865–877.

International Diabetes Federation. 2009. Diabetes Atlas, 4th Edition. (http://www.idf.org)

Ipp E, Dobbs RE, Arimura A, Vale W, Harris V, Unger RH. 1977. Release of immunoreactive somatostatin from the pancreas in response to glucose, amino acids, pancreozymin-cholecystokinin, and tolbutamide. *J Clin Invest* 60:760–765.

Israelian Z, Gosmanov NR, Szoke E, Schorr M, Bokhari S, Cryer PE, Gerich JE, Meyer C. 2005. Increasing the decrement in intraislet insulin improves glucagon responses to hypoglycemia in advanced type 2 diabetes. *Diabetes Care* 28:2691–2696.

Itoh Y, Esaki T, Shimoji K, Cook M, Law MJ, Kaufman E, Sokoloff L. 2003. Dichloroacetate effects on glucose and lactate oxidation by neurons and astroglia in vitro and on glucose utilization by brain in vivo. *Proc Natl Acad Sci USA* 100:4879–4884.

Jacobsen AM. 1996. The psychological care of patients with insulin-dependent diabetes mellitus. *N Engl J Med* 344:1249–1253.

Jacobsen AM, Ryan CM, Cleary PA, Waberski BH, Weinger K, Musen G, Dahms W, DCCT/EDIC Research Group. 2011. Biomedical risk factors for decreased cognitive functioning in type 1 diabetes: an 18 year follow-up of the Diabetes Control and Complication Trial (DCCT) cohort. *Diabetologia* 54:245–255.

Jaferi A, Nowak N, Bhatnagar S. 2003. Negative feedback functions in chronically stressed rats: role of the posterior paraventricular thalamus. *Physiol & Behavior* 78:365–373.

Jeitler K, Horvath K, Berghold A, Gratzer TW, Neeser K, Pieber TR, Siebenhofer A. 2008. Continuous subcutaneous insulin infusion versus multiple daily injections in patients with diabetes mellitus: systematic review and meta-analysis. *Diabetologia* 51:941–951.

Johannesen J, Svensson J, Bergholdt R, Eising S, Gramstrup H, Frandsen E, Dick-Nielsen J, Hansen L, Pociot F, Mortensen HB, The Danish Society for Diabetes in Childhood and Adolescence. 2010. Hypoglycemia, S-ACE and ACE genotypes in a Danish nationwide population of children and adolescents with type 1 diabetes. *Pediatr Diabetes* 12:100–106.

Johnston SS, Conner C, Aagren M, Smith DM, Bouchard J, Brett J. 2011. Evidence linking hypoglycemic events to an increased risk of acute cardiovascular events in patients with type 2 diabetes. *Diabetes Care* 34:1164–1170.

Jones TW, Boulware SD, Kraemer DT, Caprio S, Sherwin RS, Tamborlane WV. 1991. Independent effects of youth and poor diabetes control on responses to hypoglycemia in children. *Diabetes* 40:358–363.

Jones TW, Porter P, Sherwin RS, Davis EA, O'Leary P, Frazer F, Byrne G, Stick S, Tamborlane WV. 1998. Decreased epinephrine responses to hypoglycemia during sleep. *N Engl J Med* 338:1657–1662.

Joseph SE, Heaton N, Potter D, Pernet A, Umpleby MA, Amiel SA. 2000. Renal glucose production compensates for the liver during the anhepatic phase of liver transplantation. *Diabetes* 49:450–456.

Juvenile Diabetes Research Foundation (JDRF) Continuous Glucose Monitoring Study Group. 2008. Continuous glucose monitoring and intensive treatment of type 1 diabetes. *N Engl J Med* 359:1464–1476.

———. 2009a. Factors predictive of use and of benefit from continuous glucose monitoring in type 1 diabetes. *Diabetes Care* 32:1947–1953.

————. 2009b. Sustained benefit of continuous glucose monitoring on A1C, glucose profiles, and hypoglycemia in adults with type 1 diabetes. *Diabetes Care* 32:2047–2049.

————. 2010. Prolonged nocturnal hypoglycemia is common during 12 months of continuous glucose monitoring in children and adults with type 1 diabetes. *Diabetes Care* 33:1004–1008.

Kahn KJ, Myers RE. 1971. Insulin induced hypoglycaemia in the non-human primate. I. Clinical consequences. In Brain Hypoxia. Brierley JB, Meldrum BS, Eds. London, William Heinemann Medical Books, pp. 185–194.

Kalopita S, Stathi C, Thomaskos P, Vlahodimitris I, Liatis S, Makrilakis K. 2011. Relationship of hypoglycaemia with QTc prolongation in patients with type 2 diabetes (abstract). *Diabetologia* 54(Suppl 1):S112.

Kang L, Sanders NM, Dunn-Meynell AA, Gaspers LD, Routh VH, Thomas AP, Levin BE. 2008. Prior hypoglycemia enhances glucose responsiveness in some ventromedial hypothalamic glucosensing neurons. Am J Physiol Regul Integr Comp Physiol 294:R784–R792.

Kansagara D, Fu R, Freeman M, Wolf F, Helfand M. 2011. Intensive insulin therapy in hospitalized patients. A systematic review. *Ann Intern Med* 154:268–282.

Kavanagh BP, McCowen KC. 2010. Glycemic control in the ICU. *N Engl J Med* 363:2540–2546.

Keen AJ, Duncan E, McKillop-Smith A, Evans ND, Gold AE. 2012. Dose adjustment for normal eating (DAFNE) in routine clinical practice: who benefits? *Diabet Med* 29:670–676.

Kern W, Peters A, Fruehwald-Schultes B, Deininger E, Born J, Fehm HL. 2001. Improving influence of insulin on cognitive functions in humans. *Neuroendocrinology* 74:270–280.

Kilpatrick ES, Rigby AS, Goode K, Atkin SL. 2007. Relating mean blood glucose and glucose variability to the risk of multiple episodes of hypoglycaemia in type 1 diabetes. *Diabetologia* 50:2553–2561.

Knudsen GM, Hasselbach SG, Hertz MM, Paulson OB. 1999. High dose insulin does not increase glucose transfer across the blood-brain barrier in humans: a re-evaluation. *Eur J Clin Invest* 29:687–691.

Konarska M, Stewart RE, McCarty R. 1989. Habituation of sympathetic-adrenal medullary responses following exposure to chronic intermittent stress. *Physiol Behav* 45:255–261.

Konarska M, Stewart RE, McCarty R. 1990. Predictability of chronic intermittent stress: effects on sympathetic-adrenal medullary responses of laboratory rats. *Behav Neural Biol* 53:231–243.

Kovatchev BP, Cox DJ, Gonder-Frederick LA, Young-Hyman D, Schlundt D, Clarke WL. 1998. Assessment of risk for severe hypoglycemia among adults with IDDM: validation of the low blood glucose index. *Diabetes Care* 21:1870–1875.

Kovatchev BP, Cox DJ, Kumar A, Gonder-Frederick LA, Clarke WL. 2003. Algorithmic evaluation of metabolic control and risk of severe hypoglycemia in type 1 and type 2 diabetes using self-monitoring blood glucose (SMBG) data. *Diabetes Technol Ther* 5:817–828.

Lachin JM. 2010. Intensive glycemic control and mortality in ACCORD – a chance finding? *Diabetes Care* 33:2719–2721.

Lachin JM, Genuth S, Nathan DM, Zinman B, Rutledge BN, for the DCCT/EDIC Research Group. 2008. Effect of glycemic exposure on the risk of microvascular complications in the Diabetes Control and Complication Trial— revisited. *Diabetes* 57:995–1001.

Laing SP, Swerdlow AJ, Slater SD, Botha JL, Burden AC, Waugh NR, Smith AWM, Hill RD, Bingley PJ, Patterson CC, Qiao Z, Keen H. 1999. The British Diabetic Association Cohort Study. I. All-cause mortality in patients with insulin-treated diabetes mellitus. *Diabetic Med* 16:459–465.

Laitinen T, Lyyra-Laitinen T, Huopio H, Vauhkonen I, Halonen T, Hartikainen J, Niskanen L, Laakso M. 2008. Electrocardiographic alterations during hyperinsulinemic hypoglycemia in healthy subjects. Ann Noninvasive *Electrocardiol* 13:97–105.

Langendam M, Luijf YM, Hooft L, DeVries JH, Mudde AH, Scholten RJPM. 2012. Continuous glucose monitoring systems for type 1 diabetes mellitus. Cochrane Database Syst Rev. doi: 10.1002/14651858. CD008101. pub2.

Lee S, Harris ND, Robinson RT, Yeoh L, Macdonald IA, Heller SR. 2003. Effects of adrenaline and potassium on QTc interval and QT dispersion in man. *Eur J Clin Invest* 33:93–98.

Lee SP, Harris ND, Robinson RT, Davies C, Ireland R, Macdonald IA, Heller SR. 2005. Effect of atenolol on QTc interval lengthening during hypoglycaemia in type 1 diabetes. *Diabetologia* 48:1269–1272.

Lee SP, Yeoh L, Harris ND, Davies CM, Robinson RT, Leathard A, Newman C, Macdonald IA, Heller SR. 2004. Influence of autonomic neuropathy on QTc interval lengthening during hypoglycemia in type 1 diabetes. *Diabetes* 53:1535–1542.

Lee Y, Wang M-Y, Du XQ, Charron MJ, Unger RH. 2011. Glucagon receptor knockout prevents insulin-deficient type 1 diabetes in mice. *Diabetes* 60:391–397.

Leese GP, Wang J, Broomhall J, Kelly P, Marsden A, Morrison W, Frier BM, Morris AD, DARTS/MEMO Collaboration. 2003. Frequency of severe hypoglycemia requiring emergency treatment in type 1 and type 2 diabetes: a population based study of health service resource use. *Diabetes Care* 26:1176-1180.

Leu J, Cui M-H, Shamoon H, Gabriely I. 2009. Hypoglycemia-associated autonomic failure is prevented by opioid receptor blockade. *J Clin Endocrinol Metab* 94:3372–3380.

Levin BE, Becker TC, Eiki J, Zhang BB, Dunn-Meynell AA. 2008. Ventromedial hypothalamic glucokinase is an important mediator of the counterregulatory response to insulin-induced hypoglycemia. *Diabetes* 57:1371–1379.

Levin BE, Magnan C, Dunn-Meynell A, Le Foll C. 2011. Metabolic sensing and the brain: who, what, where, and how? *Endocrinology* 152:2552–2557.

Levy CJ, Kinsley BT, Bajaj M, Simonson DC. 1998. Effect of glycemic control on glucose counterregulation during hypoglcyemia in NIDDM. *Diabetes Care* 21:1330–1338.

Little S, Shaw J, Home P. 2011. Hypoglycemia rates with basal insulin analogs. *Diabetes Technol Ther* 13 (Suppl 1):S53–S64.

Lubow JM, Piñón IG, Avogaro A, Cobelli C, Treeson DM, Mandeville KA, Toffolo G, Boyle PJ. 2006. Brain oxygen utilization is unchanged by hypoglycemia in normal humans: lactate, alanine, and leucine uptake are not sufficient to offset energy deficit. *Am J Physiol Endocrinol Metab* 290:E149–E153.

Lüddeke H-J, Sreenan S, Aczel S, Maxeiner S, Yeniqun M, Kozlovski P, Gydesen H, Dornhorst A, on behalf of the PREDICTIVE Study Group. 2007. PREDICTIVE – A global, prospective observational study to evaluate insulin detemir treatment in types 1 and 2 diabetes: baseline characteristics and predictors of hypoglycemia from the European cohort. *Diabetes Obes Metab* 9:428–434.

Ly TT, Gallego PH, Davis EA, Jones TW. 2009. Impaired awareness of hypoglycemia in a population-based sample of children and adolescents with type 1 diabetes. *Diabetes Care* 32:1802–1806.

Ly TT, Hewitt J, Davey RJ, Lim E-M, Davis EA, Jones TW. 2011. Improving epinephrine responses in hypoglycemia unawareness with real-time continuous glucose monitoring in adolescents with type 1 diabetes. *Diabetes Care* 34:50–52.

Ly TT, Nicholas JA, Retterath A, Davis EA, Jones TW. 2012. Analysis of glucose responses to automated insulin suspension with sensor-augmented pump therapy. *Diabetes Care* 35:1462–1465.

MacCuish AC. 1993. Treatment of hypoglycemia. In Diabetes and Hypoglycemia. Frier BM, Fisher BM, Eds. London, Edward Arnold, pp. 212–221.

MacDonald MJ. 1987. Post exercise late onset hypoglycemia in insulin-dependent diabetic patients. *Diabetes Care* 10:584–588.

MacGorman LR, Rizza RA, Gerich JE. 1981. Physiological concentrations of growth hormone exert insulin-like and insulin antagonistic effects on both hepatic and extra-hepatic tissues in man. *J Clin Endocrinol Metab* 53:556–559.

MacLeod KM, Hepburn DA, Frier BM. 1993. Frequency and morbidity of severe hypoglycaemia in insulin-treated diabetic patients. *Diabet Med* 10:238–245.

Maggs DG, Jacob R, Rife F, Caprio S, Tamborlane WV, Sherwin RS. 1997. Counterregulation in peripheral tissues. *Diabetes* 46:70–76.

Marker JC, Cryer PE, Clutter WE. 1992. Attenuated glucose recovery from hypoglycemia in the elderly. *Diabetes* 41:671–678.

Marker JC, Hirsch IB, Smith L, Parvin CA, Holloszy JO, Cryer PE. 1991. Catecholamines in the prevention of hypoglycemia during exercise in humans. *Am J Physiol Endocrinol Metab* 260:E705–E712.

Marty N, Dallaporta M, Thorens B. 2007. Brain glucose sensing, counterregulation and energy homeostasis. *Physiology* 22:241–251.

Maruyama H, Hisatomi A, Orci L, Grodsky GM, Unger RH. 1984. Insulin within islets is a physiologic glucagon release inhibitor. *J Clin Invest* 74:2296–2299.

Mason GF, Petersen KF, Lebon V, Rothman DL, Shulman GI. 2006. Increased brain monocarboxylic acid transport and utilization in type 1 diabetes. *Diabetes* 55:929–934.

Matschinsky FM, Zelent B, Doliba N, Li C, Vanderkooi JM, Naji A, Sarabu R, Grimsby J. 2011. Glucokinase activators for diabetes therapy. *Diabetes Care* 34 (Suppl 2):S236–S243.

Matyka KA, Wigg L, Pramming S, Stores G, Dunger DB. 1999. Cognitive function and mood after profound nocturnal hypoglycaemia in prepubertal children with conventional insulin treatment for diabetes. *Arch Dis Child* 81:138–142.

McCall AL, Fixman LB, Fleming N, Tornheim K, Chick W, Ruderman NB. 1986. Chronic hypoglycemia increases brain glucose transport. *Am J Physiol* 251:E442–E447.

McCoy R, Shah ND, Van Houton HK, Wermers RA, Smith SA. 2012. Increased mortality of patients with diabetes reporting severe hypoglycemia. *Diabetes Care*.35:1897–1901.

McCrimmon RJ, Deary IJ, Gold AE, Hepburn DA, MacLeod KM, Ewing FME, Frier BM. 2003. Symptoms reported during experimental hypoglycaemia: effect of method of induction of hypoglycaemia and of diabetes per se. *Diabet Med* 20:507–509.

McCrimmon RJ, Sherwin RS. 2010. Hypoglycemia in type 1 diabetes. *Diabetes* 59:2333–2339.

McGregor VP, Banarer S, Cryer PE. 2002. Elevated endogenous cortisol reduces autonomic neuroendocrine and symptom responses to subsequent hypoglycemia. *Am J Physiol Endocrinol Metab* 282:E770–E777.

McNay EC, Sherwin RS. 2004. Effect of recurrent hypoglycemia on spatial cognition and cognitive metabolism in normal and diabetic rats. *Diabetes* 53:418–425.

Meier JJ, Kjems LL, Veldhuis JD, Lefèbvre P, Butler PC. 2006. Postprandial suppression of glucagon secretion depends on intact pulsatile insulin secretion: further evidence for the intraislet insulin hypothesis. *Diabetes* 55:1051–1056.

Meneilly GS, Cheung E, Tuokko H. 1994. Altered responses to hypoglycemia of healthy elderly people. *J Clin Endocrinol Metab* 78:1341–1348.

Menge BA, Grüber L, Jørgensen SM, Deacon CF, Schmidt WE, Veldhuis JD, Holst JJ, Meier JJ. 2011. Loss of inverse relationship between pulsatile insulin and glucagon secretion in patients with type 2 diabetes. *Diabetes* 60:2160–2168.

Meyer C, Grossman R, Mitrakou A, Mahler R, Veneman T, Gerich J, Bretzel RG. 1998. Effects of autonomic neuropathy on counterregulation and awareness of hypoglycemia in type 1 diabetic patients. *Diabetes Care* 21:1960–1966.

Miller ME, Bonds DE, Gerstein HC, Seaquist ER, Bergenstal RM, Calles-Escandon J, Childress RD, Craven TE, Cuddihy RM, Dailey G, Feinglos MN, Ismail-Beigi F, Largay JF, O'Connor PJ, Paul T, Savage PJ, Schubart UK, Sood A, Genuth S, for the ACCORD investigators. 2010. The effects of baseline characteristics, glycaemia treatment approach, and glycated haemoglobin concentration on the risk of severe hypoglycaemia: post hoc epidemiological analysis of the ACCORD study. *BMJ* 340:b5444.

Milman S, Leu J, Shamoon H, Vele S, Gabriely I. 2012a. Opioid receptor blockade prevents exercise-associated autonomic failure in humans. *Diabetes* 61:1609–1615.

Milman S, Leu J, Shamoon H, Vele S, Gabriely I. 2012b. Magnitude of exercise-induced β-endorphin response is associated with subsequent development of altered hypoglycemia counterregulation. *J Clin Endocrinol Metab* 97:623–631.

Mitrakou A, Fanelli C, Veneman T, Perriello G, Calderone S, Platanisiotis D, Rambotti A, Raptis S, Brunetti P, Cryer P, Gerich J, Bolli G. 1993. Reversibility of unawareness of hypoglycemia in patients with insulinoma. *N Engl J Med* 329:834–839.

Mitrakou A, Ryan C, Veneman T, Mokan M, Jenssen T, Kiss I, Durrant J, Cryer P, Gerich J. 1991. Hierarchy of glycemic thresholds for counterregulatory hormone secretion, symptoms and cerebral dysfunction. *Am J Physiol Endocrinol Metab* 260:E67–E74.

Moghissi ES, Korytkowski MT, DiNardo M, Einhorn D, Hellman R, Hirsch IB, Inzucchi SE, Ismail-Beigi F, Kirkman MS, Umpierrez GE. 2009. American Association of Clinical Endocrinologists and American Diabetes Association consensus statement on inpatient glycemic control. *Diabetes Care* 32:1119–1131.

Mühlhauser I, Overmann H, Bender R, Bott U, Berger M. 1997. Risk factors for severe hypoglycaemia in adult patients with type 1 diabetes—a prospective population based study. *Diabetologia* 41:1274–1282.

Mukhopadhyay A, Farrell T, Fraser RB, Ola B. 2007. Continuous subcutaneous insulin infusion vs intensive conventional insulin therapy in pregnant diabetic women: a systematic review and metaanalysis of randomized, controlled trials. *Am J Obstet Gynecol* 197:447–456.

Mundinger TO, Mei Q, Figlewicz DP, Lernmark A, Taborsky GJ Jr. 2003. Impaired glucagon response to sympathetic nerve stimulation in the BB diabetic rat: effect of early sympathetic islet neuropathy. *Am J Physiol Endocrinol Metab* 285:E1047–E1054.

Murad MH, Coto-Yglesias F, Wang AT, Sheidaee N, Mullan RJ, Elamin MB, Erwin PJ, Montori VM. 2009. Drug-induced hypoglycemia: a systemic review. *J Clin Endocrinol Metab* 94:741–745.

Murata GH, Duckworth WC, Shah JH, Wendel CS, Mohler MJ, Hoffman RM. 2005. Hypoglycemia in stable, insulin-treated veterans with type 2 diabetes: a prospective study of 1662 episodes. *J Diabetes Complications* 19:10–17.

Murphy HR, Elleri D, Allen JM, Harris J, Simmons D, Rayman G, Temple R, Dunger DB, Haidar A, Nodale M, Wilinska ME, Hovorka R. 2011. Closed-loop insulin delivery during pregnancy complicated by type 1 diabetes. *Diabetes Care* 34:406–411.

Murphy NP, Ford-Adams ME, Ong KK, Harris ND, Keane SM, Davies C, Ireland RH, Macdonald IA, Knight EJ, Edge JA, Heller SR, Dunger DB. 2004. Prolonged cardiac repolarisation during spontaneous nocturnal hypoglycaemia in children and adolescents with type 1 diabetes. *Diabetologia* 47:1940–1947.

Mutel E, Gautier-Stein A, Abdul-Wahed A, Amigó-Correig M, Zitoun C, Stefanutti A, Houberdon I, Tourette JA, Mithieux G, Rajas F. 2011. Control of blood glucose in the absence of hepatic glucose production during prolonged fasting in mice. *Diabetes* 60:3121–3131.

Nehlig A. 2004. Brain uptake and metabolism of ketone bodies in animal models. *Prostaglandins Leukot Essent Fatty Acids* 70:265–275.

Nielsen LR, Pedersen-Bjergaard U, Thorsteinsson B, Johansen M, Damm P, Mathiesen ER. 2008. Hypoglycemia in pregnant women with type 1 diabetes. *Diabetes Care* 31:9–14.

Nordfeldt S, Ludvigsson J. 2005. Fear and other disturbances of severe hypoglycaemia in children and adolescents with type 1 diabetes mellitus. *J Pediatr Endocrinol Metab* 18:83–91.

Nordfeldt S, Samuelsson U. 2003. Serum ACE predicts severe hypoglycemia in children and adolescents with type 1 diabetes. *Diabetes Care* 26:274–278.

Nordin C. 2010. The case for hypoglycaemia as a proarrhythmic event: basic and clinical evidence. *Diabetologia* 53:1552–1561.

The Normoglycemia in Intensive Care Evaluation—Survival Using Glucose Algorithm Regulation [NICE-SUGAR] Study Investigators. 2009. Intensive versus conventional glucose control in critically ill patients. *N Engl J Med* 360:1283–1297.

Northam EA, Anderson PJ, Jacobs R, Hughes M, Warne GL, Werther GA. 2001. Neuropsychological profiles of children with type 1 diabetes 6 years after disease onset. *Diabetes Care* 24:1541–1546.

Northam EA, Rankins D, Lin A, Wellard RM, Pell GS, Finch SJ, Werther GA, Cameron FJ. 2009. Central nervous system function in youth with type 1 diabetes 12 years after disease onset. *Diabetes Care* 32:445–450.

Obici S, Zhang BB, Karkanias G, Rossetti L. 2002. Hypothalamic insulin signaling is required for inhibition of glucose production. *Nat Med* 8:1376–1382.

Ohkubo Y, Kishikawa H, Araki E, Miyata T, Isami S, Motoyoshi S, Kojima Y, Furuyoshi N, Shichiri M. 1995. Intensive insulin therapy prevents the progression of diabetic microvascular complications in Japanese patients with non-insulin dependent diabetes mellitus: a randomized prospective 6-year study. *Diabetes Res Clin Pract* 28:103–117.

Olsen HL, Theander S, Bokvist K, Buschard K, Wollheim CB, Gromada J. 2005. Glucose stimulates glucose release in single rat α-cells by mechanisms that mirror the stimulus-secretion coupling in β-cells. *Endocrinology* 146:4861–4870.

Osadchii OE. 2010. Mechanisms of hypokalemia-induced ventricular arrhythmogenicity. *Fundam Clin Pharmacol* 24:547–559.

Osundiji MA, Hurst P, Moore SP, Markkula SP, Yueh CY, Swamy A, Hoashi S, Shaw JS, Riches CH, Heisler LK, Evans ML. 2011. Recurrent hypoglycemia increases hypothalamic glucose phosphorylation activity in rats. *Metabolism* 60:550–556.

Ovalle F, Fanelli CG, Paramore DS, Hershey T, Craft S, Cryer PE. 1998. Brief twice-weekly episodes of hypoglycemia reduce detection of clinical hypoglycemia in type 1 diabetes mellitus. *Diabetes* 47:1472–1479.

Owen OE, Felig P, Morgan AP, Wahren J, Cahill GF. 1969. Liver and kidney metabolism during prolonged starvation. *J Clin Invest* 48:574–583.

Öz G, Seaquist ER, Kumar A, Criego AB, Benedict LE, Rao JP, Henry P-G, Van De Moortele P-F, Gruetter R. 2007. Human brain glycogen content and metabolism: implications on its role in brain energy metabolism. *Am J Physiol Endocrinol Metab* 292:E946–E951.

Öz G, Tesfaye N, Kumar A, Deelchand DK, Eberly LE, Seaquist ER. 2012. Brain glycogen content and metabolism in subjects with type 1 diabetes and hypoglycemia unawareness. *J Cereb Blood Flow Metab* 32:256–263.

Palmer JP, Henry DP, Benson JW, Johnson DG, Ensinck JW. 1976. Glucagon response to hypoglycemia in sympathectomized man. *J Clin Invest* 57:522–525.

Pankowska E, Blazik M, Dziechciarz P, Szypowska A, Szajewska H. 2009. Continuous subcutaneous insulin infusion vs. multiple daily injections in children with type 1 diabetes: a systematic review and meta-analysis of randomized control trials. *Pediatr Diabetes* 10:52–58.

Paramore DS, Fanelli CG, Shah SD, Cryer PE. 1998. Forearm norepinephrine spillover during standing, hyperinsulinemia and hypoglycemia. *Am J Physiol Endocrinol Metab* 275:E872–E881.

Paranjape SA, Chan O, Zhu W, Horblitt AM, McNay EC, Cresswell JA, Bogan JS, McCrimmon RJ, Sherwin RS. 2010. Influence of insulin in the ventromedial hypothalamus on pancreatic glucagon secretion in vivo. *Diabetes* 59:1521–1527.

Patterson CC, Dahlquist G, Harjutsalo V, Joner G, Feltbower RG, Svensson J, Schober E, Gyürüs E, Castell C, Urbonaité B, Rosenbauer J, Iotova V, Thorsson AV, Soltész G. 2007. Early mortality in EURODIAB population-based cohorts of type 1 diabetes diagnosed in childhood since 1989. *Diabetologia* 50:2439–2442.

Pedersen-Bjergaard U, Agerholm-Larsen B, Pramming S, Hougaard P, Thorsteinsson B. 2001. Activity of angiotensin-converting enzyme and risk of severe hypoglycemia in type 1 diabetes mellitus. *Lancet* 357:1248–1253.

———. 2003. Prediction of severe hypoglycaemia by angiotensin-converting enzyme activity and genotype in type 1 diabetes. *Diabetologia* 46:89–96.

Pedersen-Bjergaard U, Høi-Hansen T, Thorsteinsson B. 2007. An evaluation of methods of assessing impaired awareness of hypoglycemia in type 1 diabetes. *Diabetes Care* 30:e112.

Pedersen-Bjergaard U, Nielsen SL, Akram K, Perrild H, Nordestgaard BG, Montgomery HE, Pramming S, Thorsteinsson B. 2009. Angiotensin converting enzyme and angiotensin II receptor subtype 2 genotypes in type 1 diabetes and severe hypoglycaemia requiring emergency treatment: a case cohort study. *Pharmacogenet Genomics* 19:864–868.

Pedersen-Bjergaard U, Pramming S, Thorsteinsson B. 2003. Recall of severe hypoglycemia and self-estimated state of awareness in type 1 diabetes. *Diabetes Metab Res Rev* 19:232–240.

Pedersen-Bjergaard U, Thomsen CE, Høgenhaven H, Smed A, Kjær TW, Holst JJ, Dela F, Hilsted L, Frandsen E, Pramming S, Thorsteinsson B. 2008. Angiotensin-converting enzyme activity and cognitive impairment during hypoglycaemia in healthy humans. *JRAAS* 9:37–48.

Perantie DC, Koller JM, Weaver PM, Lugar HM, Black KJ, White NH, Hershey T. 2011. Prospectively determined impact of type 1 diabetes on brain volume during development. *Diabetes* 60:3006–3014.

Perantie DC, Wu J, Koller JM, Lim A, Warren SL, Black KJ, Sadler M, White NH, Hershey T. 2007. Regional brain volume differences associated with hyperglycemia and severe hypoglycemia in youth with type 1 diabetes. *Diabetes Care* 30:2331–2337.

Perriello G, De Feo P, Torlone E, Fanelli C, Santeusanio F, Brunetti P, Bolli GB. 1991. The dawn phenomenon in type 1 (insulin-dependent) diabetes mellitus: magnitude, frequency, variability, and dependency on glucose counter-regulation and insulin sensitivity. *Diabetologia* 34:21–28.

Pfister R, Sharp SJ, Luben R, Khaw KT, Wareham NJ. 2011. No evidence of an increased mortality risk associated with low levels of glycated haemoglobin in a non-diabetic UK population. *Diabetologia* 54:2025–2032.

Phung OJ, Scholle JM, Talwar M, Coleman CI. 2010. Effect of noninsulin antidiabetic drugs added to metformin therapy on glycemic control, weight gain and hypoglycemia in type 2 diabetes. *JAMA* 303:1410–1418.

Polak JF, Backlund J-Y, Cleary PA, Harrington AP, O'Leary DH, Lachin JM, Nathan DM, for the DCCT/EDIC Research Group. 2011. Progression of carotid artery intima-media thickness during 12 years in the Diabetes Control and Complications Trial/Epidemiology of Diabetes Interventions and Complications (DCCT/EDIC) Study. *Diabetes* 60:607–613.

Polonsky KS, Licinio-Paixao J, Given BD, Pugh W, Rue P, Galloway J, Karrison T, Frank B. 1986. Use of biosynthetic human C-peptide in the measurement of insulin secretion rates in normal volunteers and type I diabetic patients. *J Clin Invest* 77:98–105.

Porte D Jr, Baskin DG, Schwartz MW. 2005. Insulin signaling in the central nervous system: a critical role in metabolic homeostasis and disease from C. elegans to humans. *Diabetes* 54:1264–1276.

Pramming S, Thorsteinsson B, Bendtson I, Binder C. 1991. Symptomatic hypoglycaemia in 411 type 1 diabetic patients. *Diabet Med* 8:217–222.

Preiser J-C, Devos P. 2007. Clinical experience with tight glucose control by intensive insulin therapy. *Crit Care Med* 35 (Suppl 9):S503–S507.

Puente EC, Silverstein J, Bree AJ, Musikantow DR, Wozniak DF, Maloney S, Daphna-Iken D, Fisher SJ. 2010. Recurrent moderate hypoglycemia ameliorates brain damage and cognitive dysfunction induced by severe hypoglycemia. *Diabetes* 59:1055–1062.

Qaseem A, Vijan S, Snow V, Cross JT, Weiss KB, Owens DK, for the Clinical Efficacy Assessment Subcommittee of the American College of Physicians. 2007. Glycemic control and type 2 diabetes mellitus: the optimal hemoglobin A_{1C} targets: a guidance statement from the American College of Physicians. *Ann Intern Med* 147:417–422.

Quilliam BJ, Simeone JC, Ozbay AB, Kogut SJ. 2011. The incidence and costs of hypoglycemia in type 2 diabetes. *Am J Manag Care* 17:673–680.

Raju B, Arbeláez AM, Breckenridge SM, Cryer PE. 2006. Nocturnal hypoglycemia in type 1 diabetes: an assessment of preventive bedtime treatments. *J Clin Endocrinol Metab* 91:2087–2092.

Raju B, Cryer PE. 2005. Loss of the decrement in intraislet insulin plausibly explains loss of the glucagon response to hypoglycemia in insulin-deficient diabetes. *Diabetes* 54:757–764.

Raju B, McGregor VP, Cryer PE. 2003. Cortisol elevations comparable to those that occur during hypoglycemia do not cause hypoglycemia-associated autonomic failure. *Diabetes* 52:2083–2089.

Ramanathan RP, Cryer PE. 2011. Adrenergic mediation of hypoglycemia-associated autonomic failure. *Diabetes* 60:602–606.

Ramnanan CJ, Edgerton DS, Kraft G, Cherrington AD. 2011a. Physiologic action of glucagon on liver glucose metabolism. *Diabetes Obes Metab* 13(Suppl 1):118–125.

Ramnanan CJ, Saraswathi V, Smith MS, Donahue EP, Farmer B, Farmer TD, Neal D, Williams PE, Lautz M, Mari A, Cherrington AD, Edgerton DS. 2011b. Brain insulin action augments hepatic glycogen synthesis without suppressing glucose production or gluconeogenesis in dogs. *J Clin Invest* 121:3713–3723.

Redelmeier DA, Kenshole AB, Ray JG. 2009. Motor vehicle crashes in diabetic patients with tight glycemic control: a population-based case control analysis. *PLOS Medicine* 6:e1000192.

Reichard P, Pihl M. 1994. Mortality and treatment side-effects during long-term intensified conventional insulin treatment in the Stockholm Diabetes Intervention Study. *Diabetes* 43:313–317.

Reno CM, Daphna-Iken D, Fisher SJ. 2012. Adrenergic blockade prevents life threatening cardiac arrhythmias and sudden death due to severe hypoglycemia (abstract). *Diabetes* 61:A46.

Reno CM, Tanoli T, Puente EC, Bree AJ, Cui C, Silverstein J, Daphna-Iken D, Fisher SJ. 2011. Deaths due to severe hypoglycemia are exacerbated by diabetes and ameliorated by hypoglycemia pre-conditioning (abstract). *Diabetes* 60:A81.

Rickels MR. 2012. Recovery of endocrine function after islet and pancreas transplantation. *Curr Diab Rep.* doi: 10.1007/s11892–012–0294–3.

Rickels MR, Cullison K, Fuller C, Dalton-Bakes C, Markmann E, Palanjian M, Liu C, Kapoor S, Teff KL, Naji A. 2011. Improvement of glucose counterregulation following human islet transplantation in long-standing type 1 diabetes: preliminary results (abstract). *Diabetes* 60:A80.

Rickels MR, Schutta MH, Mueller R, Kapoor S, Markmann JF, Naji A, Teff KL. 2007. Glycemic thresholds for activation of counterregulatory hormone and symptom responses in islet transplant recipients. *J Clin Endocrinol Metab* 92:873–879.

Ricks J, Molnar MZ, Kovesdy CP, Shah A, Nissenson AR, Williams M, Kalantar-Zadeh K. 2012. Glycemic control and cardiovascular mortality in hemodialysis patients with diabetes. *Diabetes* 61:708–715.

Riddle MC. 2010. Intensive glucose control and mortality in ACCORD – still looking for clues. *Diabetes Care* 33:2722–2724.

Riddle MC, Ambrosius WT, Brillon DJ, Buse JB, Byington RP, Cohen RM, Goff DC Jr, Malozowski S, Margolis KL, Probstfield JL, Schnall A, Seaquist ER, for the Action to Control Cardiovascular Risk in Diabetes Investigators. 2010. Epidemiologic relationships between A1C and all-cause mortality during a median 3.4-year follow-up of glycemic treatment in the ACCORD trial. *Diabetes Care* 33:983–990.

Rivera N, Ramnanan CJ, An Z, Farmer T, Smith M, Farmer B, Irimia JM, Snead W, Lautz M, Roach PJ, Cherrington AD. 2010. Insulin-induced hypoglycemia increases hepatic sensitivity to glucagon in dogs. *J Clin Invest* 120:4425–4435.

Rizza RA, Cryer PE, Gerich JE. 1979. Role of glucagon, catecholamines, and growth hormone in human glucose counterregulation. *J Clin Invest* 64:62–71.

Rizza RA, Cryer PE, Haymond MW, Gerich JE. 1980. Adrenergic mechanisms for the effect of epinephrine on glucose production and clearance in man. *J Clin Invest* 65:682–689.

Rizza RA, Mandarino L, Gerich J. 1982. Cortisol-induced insulin resistance in man: impaired suppression of glucose production and stimulation of glucose utilization due to a post-receptor defect of insulin action. *J Clin Endocrinol Metab* 54:131–138.

Robertson H, Pearson DWM, Gold AE. 2009. Severe hypoglycaemia during pregnancy in women with type 1 diabetes is common and planning pregnancy does not decrease the risk. *Diabet Med* 26:824–826.

Robinson RT, Harris ND, Ireland RH, Lee S, Newman C, Heller SR. 2003. Mechanisms of abnormal cardiac repolarization during insulin-induced hypoglycemia. *Diabetes* 52:1469–1474.

Robinson RT, Harris ND, Ireland RH, Macdonald IA, Heller SR. 2004. Changes in cardiac repolarization during clinical episodes of nocturnal hypoglycaemia in adults with type 1 diabetes. *Diabetologia* 47:312–315.

Rosen SG, Clutter WE, Berk MA, Shah SD, Cryer PE. 1984. Epinephrine supports the postabsorptive plasma glucose concentration and prevents hypoglycemia when glucagon secretion is deficient in man. *J Clin Invest* 73:405–411.

Rosenn BM, Miodovnik M, Khoury JC, Siddiqi TA. 1996. Counterregulatory hormonal responses to hypoglycemia during pregnancy. *Obstet Gynecol* 87:568–574.

Rossetti P, Porcellati F, Bolli GB, Fanelli CG. 2008. Prevention of hypoglycemia while achieving good glycemic control in type 1 diabetes. *Diabetes Care* 31 (Suppl 2):S113–S120.

Rossetti P, Porcellati F, Busciantella Ricci N, Candeloro P, Cioli P, Nair KS, Santeusanio F, Bolli GB, Fanelli CG. 2008. Effect of oral amino acids on counterregulatory responses and cognitive function during insulin-induced hypoglycemia in nondiabetic and type 1 diabetic people. *Diabetes* 57:1905–1917.

Ruegemer JJ, Squires RW, Marsh HM, Haymond MW, Cryer PE, Rizza RA, Miles JM. 1990. Differences between prebreakfast and late afternoon glycemic responses to exercise in IDDM patients. *Diabetes Care* 13:104–110.

Ryder REJ, Owens DR, Hayes TM, Ghatei MA, Bloom SR. 1990. Unawareness of hypoglycaemia and inadequate hypoglycaemic counterregulation: no causal relation with diabetic autonomic neuropathy. *BMJ* 301:783–787.

Samols E, Stagner JI, Ewart RBL, Marks V. 1988. The order of islet microvascular cellular perfusion is B–A–D in the perfused rat pancreas. *J Clin Invest* 82:350–353.

Samols E, Tyler J, Marks V. 1972. Glucagon-insulin interrelationships. In *Glucagon: Molecular Physiology, Clinical and Therapeutic Implications*. Lefebvre P, Unger RH, Eds. Elmsford, N.Y., Pergamon Press, pp. 151–174.

Sanders NM, Wilkinson CW, Taborsky GJ Jr, Al-Noori S, Daumen W, Zavosh A, Figlewicz DP. 2008. The selective serotonin reuptake inhibitor sertraline enhances counterregulatory responses to hypoglycemia. *Am J Physiol Endocrinol Metab* 294:E853–E860.

Sandoval DA, Aftab Guy DL, Richardson MA, Ertl AC, Davis SN. 2004. Effects of low and moderate antecedent exercise on counterregulatory responses to subsequent hypoglycemia in type 1 diabetes. *Diabetes* 53:1798–1806.

Saudek CD, Duckworth WC, Giobbie-Hurder A, Henderson WG, Henry RR, Kelley DE, Edelman SV, Zieve FJ, Adler RA, Anderson JW, Anderson RJ, Hamilton BP, Donner TW, Kirkman MS, Morgan NA. 1996. Implantable insulin pump vs. multiple dose insulin for non-insulin dependent diabetes mellitus: a randomized clinical trial. *JAMA* 276:1322–1327.

Schopman JE, Geddes J, Frier BM. 2010. Prevalence of impaired awareness of hypoglycaemia and frequency of hypoglycaemia in insulin-treated type 2 diabetes. *Diabetes Res Clin Pract* 87:64–68.

————. 2011. Frequency of symptomatic and asymptomatic hypoglycaemia in type 1 diabetes: effect of impaired awareness of hypoglycaemia. *Diabet Med* 28:352–355.

Schouwenberg BJJ, Smits P, Tack CJ, de Galan BE. 2011. The effect of antecedent hypoglycaemia on β_2-adrenergic sensitivity in healthy participants with the Arg16Gly polymorphism of the β2-adrenergic receptor. *Diabetologia* 54:1212–1218.

Schramm TK, Gislason GH, Vaag A, Rasmussen JN, Folke F, Hansen ML, Fosbøl EL, Køber L, Norgaard ML, Madsen M, Hansen PR, Torp-Pedersen C. 2011. Mortality and cardiovascular risk associated with different insulin secretagogues compared with metformin in type 2 diabetes, with or without a previous myocardial infarction: a nationwide study. *Eur Heart J* 32:1900–1908.

Schultes B, Jauch-Chara K, Gais S, Hallschmid M, Reiprich E, Kern W, Oltmanns KM, Peters A, Fehm HL, Born J. 2007. Defective awakening response to nocturnal hypoglycemia in patients with type 1 diabetes mellitus. *PLoS Medicine* 4:e69.

Schultes B, Oltmanns KM, Kern W, Fehm HL, Born J, Peters A. 2003. Modulation of hunger by plasma glucose and metformin. *J Clin Endocrinol Metab* 88:1133-1141.

Schwartz NS, Clutter WE, Shah SD, Cryer PE. 1987. Glycemic thresholds for activation of glucose counterregulatory systems are higher than the threshold for symptoms. *J Clin Invest* 79:777-781.

Seaquist ER, Damberg GS, Tkac I, Gruetter R. 2001. The effect of insulin on in vivo cerebral glucose concentrations and rates of glucose transport/metabolism in humans. *Diabetes* 50:2203-2209.

Segel SA, Fanelli CG, Dence CS, Markham J, Videen TO, Paramore DS, Powers WJ, Cryer PE. 2001. Blood-to-brain glucose transport, cerebral glucose metabolism and cerebral blood flow are not increased following hypoglycemia. *Diabetes* 50:1911-1917.

Segel SA, Paramore DS, Cryer PE. 2002. Hypoglycemia-associated autonomic failure in advanced type 2 diabetes. *Diabetes* 51:724-733.

Service FJ, Rizza RA, Zimmerman BR, Dyck PJ, O'Brien PC, Melton LJ III. 1997. The classification of diabetes by clinical and C-peptide criteria. *Diabetes Care* 20:198–201.

Selvin E, Steffes MW, Zhu H, Matsushita K, Wagenknecht L, Pankow J, Coresh J, Brancati FL. 2010. Glycated hemoglobin, diabetes, and cardiovascular risk in nondiabetic adults. *N Engl J Med* 362:800–811.

Sherck SM, Shiota M, Saccomando J, Cardin S, Allen EJ, Hastings JR, Neal DW, Williams PE, Cherrington AD. 2001. Pancreatic response to mild non-insulin induced hypoglycemia does not involve extrinsic neural input. *Diabetes* 50:2487–2496.

Sherwin RS. 2008. Bringing light to the dark side of diabetes. A journey across the blood-brain barrier. *Diabetes* 57:2259–2267.

Shurraw S, Hemmelgarn B, Lin M, Majumdar SR, Klarenbach S, Manns B, Bello A, James M, Turin TC, Tonelli T for the Alberta Kidney Disease Network. 2011. Association between glycemic control and adverse outcomes in people with diabetes mellitus and chronic kidney disease. *Arch Intern Med* 171:1920–1927.

Siebenhofer A, Plank J, Berghold A, Jeitler K, Horvath K, Narath M, Gfrerer R, Pieber TR. 2006. Short acting insulin analogues versus regular human insulin in patients with diabetes mellitus. *Cochrane Database Syst Rev Apr* 19;(2):CD003287.

Simpson IA, Appel NM, Hokari M, Oki J, Holman GD, Maher F, Koehler-Stec EM, Vannucci SJ, Smith QR. 1999. Blood-brain barrier glucose transporter: effects of hypo- and hyperglycemia revisited. *J Neurochem* 72:238–247.

Sjöbom NC, Adamson U, Lins P-E. 1989. The prevalence of impaired glucose counter-regulation during an insulin infusion test in insulin-treated diabetic patients prone to severe hypoglycaemia. Diabetologia 32:818–825.

Skrivarhaug T, Bangstad H-J, Stene LC, Sandvik L, Hanssen KF, Joner G. 2006. Long-term mortality in a nationwide cohort of childhood-onset type 1 diabetic patients in Norway. *Diabetologia* 49:298–305.

Skyler JS. 2010. Glycemia and cardiovascular diseases in type 2 diabetes. *J Intern Med* 268:468–470.

Spyer G, Hattersley AT, Macdonald IA, Amiel S, MacLeod KM. 2000. Hypoglycaemic counter-regulation at normal blood glucose concentrations in patients with well controlled type-2 diabetes. *Lancet* 356:1970–1974.

Steffes MW, Sibley S, Jackson M, Thomas W. 2003. β-Cell function and the development of diabetes related complications in the Diabetes Control and Complications Trial. *Diabetes Care* 26:832–836.

Stettler C, Allemann S, Jüni P, Cull CA, Holman RR, Egger M, Krähenbühl S, Diem P. 2006. Glycemic control and macrovascular disease in types 1 and 2 diabetes: meta-analysis of randomized trials. *Am Heart J* 152:27–38.

Suh SW, Aoyama K, Chen Y, Garnier P, Matsumori Y, Gum E, Liu J, Swanson RA. 2003. Hypoglycemic neuronal death and cognitive impairment are prevented by poly(ADP-ribose) polymerase inhibitors administered after hypoglycemia. *J Neurosci* 23:10681–10690.

Suh SW, Gum ET, Hamby AM, Chan PH, Swanson RA. 2007b. Hypoglycemic neuronal death is triggered by glucose reperfusion and activation of neuronal NADPH oxidase. *J Clin Invest* 117:910–918.

Suh SW, Hamby AM, Swanson RA. 2007a. Hypoglycemia, brain energetic and hypoglycemic neuronal death. *GLIA* 55:1280–1286.

Szepietowska B, Zhu W, Chan O, Horblitt A, Dziura J, Sherwin RS. 2011. Modulation of β-adrenergic receptors in the ventromedial hypothalamus influences counterregulatory responses to hypoglycemia. *Diabetes* 60:3154–3158.

Taborsky GJ Jr, Ahrén B, Havel PJ. 1998. Autonomic mediation of glucagon secretion during hypoglycemia. *Diabetes* 47:995–1005.

Taborsky GJ Jr, Mei Q, Hackney DJ, Figlewicz DP, LeBoeuf R, Mundinger TO. 2009. Loss of islet sympathetic nerves and impairment of glucagon secretion in the NOD mouse: relationship to invasive insulitis. *Diabetologia* 52:2602–2611.

Tanenberg RJ, Newton CA, Drake AJ III. 2010. Confirmation of hypoglycemia in the "dead-in-bed" syndrome, as captured by a retrospective continuous glucose monitoring system. *Endocr Pract* 16:244–248.

Tansey MJ, Tsalikian E, Beck RW, Mauras N, Buckingham BA, Weinzimer SA, Janz KF, Kollman C, Xing D, Ruedy KJ, Steffes MW, Borland TM, Singh RJ, Tamborlane WV, for the Diabetes Research in Children Network (DirecNet) Study Group. 2006. The effects of aerobic exercise on glucose and counterregulatory hormone concentrations in children with type 1 diabetes. *Diabetes Care* 29:20–25.

Taplin CE, Cobry E, Messer L, McFann K, Chase HP, Fiallo-Scharer R. 2010. Preventing post-exercise nocturnal hypoglycemia in children with type 1 diabetes. *J Pediatr* 157:784–788.

Teh MM, Dunn JT, Choudhary P, Samarasinghe Y, Macdonald I, O'Doherty M, Marsden P, Reed LJ, Amiel SA. 2010. Evolution and resolution of human brain perfusion responses to the stress of induced hypoglycemia. *NeuroImage* 53:584–592.

Tesfaye N, Mangia S, De Martino F, Kumar A, Moheet A, Iverson E, Eberly LE, Seaquist ER. 2011. Hypoglycemia induced increases in cerebral blood flow are blunted in subjects with type 1 diabetes and hypoglycemia unawareness (abstract). *Diabetes* 60:A79.

Teves D, Videen TO, Cryer PE, Powers WJ. 2004. Activation of human medial prefrontal cortex during autonomic responses to hypoglycemia. *Proc Natl Acad Sci U S A* 101:6217–6221.

Tong Q, Ye CP, McCrimmon RJ, Dhillon H, Choi B, Kramer MD, Yu J, Yang Z, Christiansen LM, Lee CE, Choi CS, Zigman JM, Shulman GI, Sherwin RS, Elmquist JK, Lowell BB. 2007. Synaptic glutamate release by ventromedial hypothalamic neurons is part of the neurocircuitry that prevents hypoglycemia. *Cell Metab* 5:383–393.

Tordjman KM, Havlin CE, Levandoski LA, White NH, Santiago JV, Cryer PE. 1987. Failure of nocturnal hypoglycemia to cause fasting hyperglycemia in patients with insulin-dependent diabetes mellitus. *N Engl J Med* 317:1552–1559.

Towler DA, Havlin CE, Craft S, Cryer PE. 1993. Mechanism of awareness of hypoglycemia: perception of neurogenic (predominantly cholinergic) rather than neuroglycopenic symptoms. *Diabetes* 42:1791–1798.

Tsalikian E, Mauras N, Beck RW, Tamborlane WV, Janz KF, Chase HP, Wysocki T, Weinzimer SA, Buckingham BA, Kollman C, Xing D, Ruedy KJ, for the Diabetes Research in Network (DirecNet) Study Group. 2005. Impact of exercise on overnight glycemic control in children with type 1 diabetes. *J Pediatr* 147:528–534.

Tschope D, Bramlage P, Binz C, Krekler M, Plate T, Deeg E, Gitt AK. 2011. Antidiabetic pharmacotherapy and anamnestic hypoglycemia in a large cohort of type 2 diabetic patients - an analysis of the DiaRegis registry. *Cardiovasc Diabetol* 10:66.

Tse TF, Clutter WE, Shah SD, Cryer PE. 1983a. Mechanisms of postprandial glucose counterregulation in man: physiologic roles of glucagon and epinephrine vis-à-vis insulin in the prevention of hypoglycemia late after glucose ingestion. *J Clin Invest* 72:278–286.

Tse TF, Clutter WE, Shah SD, Miller JP, Cryer PE. 1983b. Neuroendocrine responses to glucose ingestion in man: specificity, temporal relationships and quantitative aspects. *J Clin Invest* 72:270–277.

Tunbridge WMG. 1981. Factors contributing to deaths of diabetics under 50 years of age. *Lancet* 2:569–572.

Turner BC, Jenkins E, Kerr D, Sherwin RS, Cavan DA. 2001. The effect of evening alcohol consumption on next-morning glucose control in type 1 diabetes. *Diabetes Care* 24:1888–1893.

Turner RC, Cull CA, Frighi V, Holman RR, UK Prospective Diabetes Study (UKPDS) Group. 1999. Glycemic control with diet, sulfonylurea, metformin, or insulin in patients with type 2 diabetes mellitus: progressive requirement for multiple therapies (UKPDS 49). *JAMA* 281:2005–2012.

U.K. Hypoglycaemia Study Group [UK Hypo Group]. 2007. Risk of hypoglycaemia in types 1 and 2 diabetes: effects of treatment modalities and their duration. *Diabetologia* 50:1140–1147.

U.K. Prospective Diabetes Study Group [UKPDS]. 1995. Overview of 6 years of therapy of type II diabetes: a progressive disease. *Diabetes* 44:1249–1258.

———. 1998a. Intensive blood-glucose control with sulphonylureas or insulin compared with conventional treatment and risk of complications in patients with type 2 diabetes (UKPDS 33). *Lancet* 352:837–853.

———. 1998b. Effect of intensive blood-glucose control with metformin on complications in overweight patients with type 2 diabetes (UKPDS 34). *Lancet* 352:854–865.

———. 1998c. United Kingdom Prospective Diabetes Study 24: a six year, randomized, controlled trial comparing sulfonylurea, insulin and metformin therapy in patients with newly diagnosed type 2 diabetes that could not be controlled with diet therapy. *Ann Intern Med* 128:165–175.

Unger RH, Orci L. 1975. The essential role of glucagon in the pathogenesis of diabetes mellitus. *Lancet* 1:14–16.

Vallbo AB, Hagbarth K-E, Wallin BG. 2004. Microneurography: how the technique developed and its role in the investigation of the sympathetic nervous system. *J Appl Physiol* 96:1262–1269.

van de Ven KCC, de Galan BE, van der Graaf M, Shestov AA, Henry P-G, Tack CJJ, Heerschap A. 2011. Effect of acute hypoglycemia on human cerebral glucose metabolism measured by ^{13}C magnetic resonance spectroscopy. *Diabetes* 60:1467–1473.

van Hall G, Strømstad M, Rasmussen P, Jans Ø, Zaar M, Gam C, Quistorff B, Secher NH, Nielsen HB. 2009. Blood lactate is an important energy source for the human brain. *J Cereb Blood Flow Metab* 29:1121–1129.

Vele S, Milman S, Shamoon H, Gabriely I. 2011. Opioid receptor blockade improves hypoglycemia-associated autonomic failure in type 1 diabetes mellitus. *J Clin Endocrinol Metab* 96:3424–3431.

Wahren J, Ekberg K, Fernqvist-Forbes E, Nair S. 1999. Brain substrate utilization during acute hypoglycaemia. *Diabetologia* 42:812–818.

Walker JN, Ramracheya R, Zhang Q, Johnson PRV, Braun M, Rorsman P. 2011. Regulation of glucagon secretion by glucose: paracrine, intrinsic or both? *Diabetes Obes Metab* 13(Suppl 1):95–105.

Watts AG, Donovan CM. 2010. Sweet talk in the brain: glucosensing, neural networks, and hypoglycemic counterregulation. *Front Neuroendocrinol* 31:32–43.

Weinberg MS, Johnson DC, Bhatt AP, Spencer RL. 2010. Medial prefrontal cortex activity can disrupt the expression of stress response habituation. *Neuroscience* 168:744–756.

Whipple AO. 1938. The surgical therapy of hyperinsulinism. *J Int Chir* 3:237–276.

White NH, Skor DA, Cryer PE, Levandoski LA, Bier DM, Santiago JV. 1983. Identification of type 1 diabetic patients at increased risk for hypoglycemia during intensive therapy. *N Engl J Med* 308:485–491.

Whitmer RA, Karter AJ, Yaffe K, Quesenberry CP Jr, Selby JV. 2009. Hypoglycemic episodes and risk of dementia in older patients with type 2 diabetes mellitus. *JAMA* 301:1565–1572.

Wiethop BV, Cryer PE. 1993a. Glycemic actions of alanine and terbutaline in IDDM. *Diabetes Care* 16:1124–1130.

———. 1993b. Alanine and terbutaline in the treatment of hypoglycemia in IDDM. *Diabetes Care* 16:1131–1136.

Wild D, von Maltzahn R, Brohan E, Christensen T, Clausen P, Gonder-Frederick L. 2007. A critical review of the literature on fear of hypoglycemia in diabetes: implications for diabetes management and patient education. *Patient Educ Couns* 68:10–15.

Wilinska ME, Budiman ES, Taub MB, Elleri D, Allen JM, Acerini CL, Dunger DB, Hovorka R. 2009. Overnight closed-loop insulin delivery with model predictive control: assessment of hypoglycemia and hyperglycemia risk using simulation studies. *J Diabetes Sci Technol* 3:1109–1120.

Witsch J, Neugebauer H, Flechsenhar J, Jüttler E. 2012. Hypoglycemic encephalopathy: a case series and literature review on outcome determination. *J Neurol.* doi: 10.1007/s00415-012-6480-z.

Won SJ, Jang BG, Yoo BH, Sohn M, Lee MW, Choi BY, Kim JH, Song HK, Suh SW. 2012. Prevention of acute/severe hypoglycemia-induced neuron death by lactate administration. *J Cereb Blood Flow Metab* 32:1086–1096.

Wright AD, Cull CA, MacLeod KM, Holman RR, for the UKPDS Group. 2006. Hypoglycemia in type 2 diabetic patients randomized to and maintained on monotherapy with diet, sulfonylurea, metformin, or insulin for 6 years from diagnosis: UKPDS 73. *J Diabetes Complications* 20:395–401.

Wurtman RJ. 2002. Stress and the adrenocortical control of epinephrine synthesis. *Metabolism* 51:11–14.

Wurtman RJ, Axelrod J. 1965. Adrenaline synthesis: control by the pituitary gland and adrenal glucocorticoids. *Science* 150:1464–1465.

Yeh H-C, Brown TT, Maruthur N, Ranasinghe P, Berger Z, Suh YD, Wilson LM, Haberl EB, Brick J, Bass EB, Golden SH. 2012. Comparative effectiveness and safety of methods of insulin delivery and glucose monitoring for diabetes mellitus: a systematic review and meta-analysis. *Ann Intern Med.* doi: 10.7326/0003–4819–157–5–201209040–00508

Yki-Järvinen H, Ryysy L, Nikkilä K, Tulokas T, Vanamo R, Heikkilä M. 1999. Comparison of bedtime insulin regimens in patients with type 2 diabetes mellitus. *Ann Intern Med* 130:389–396.

Younk LM, Davis SN. 2011. Hypoglycemia and vascular disease. *Clin Chem* 57:258–260.

Yu JTY, Burdett E, Coy DH, Giacca A, Efendic S, Vranic M. 2012. Somatostatin receptor type 2 antagonism improves glucagon and corticosterone counterregulatory responses to hypoglycemia in streptozotocin-induced diabetic rats. *Diabetes* 61:197–207.

Zammitt N, Geddes J, Warren RE, Marioni R, Ashby PJ, Frier BM. 2007. Serum angiotensin-converting enzyme and frequency of severe hypoglycaemia in type 1 diabetes: does a relationship exist? *Diabet Med* 24:1449–1454.

Zeller M, Danchin N, Simon D, Vahanian A, Lorgis L, Cottin Y, Berland J, Gueret P, Wyart P, Deturck R, Tabone X, Machecourt J, Leclercq F, Drouet E, Mulak G, Bataille V, Cambou JP, Ferrieres J, Simon T, and the French Registry of Acute ST-Elevation and Non-ST-Elevation Myocardial Infarction investigators. 2008. Impact of type of preadmission sulfonylureas on mortality and cardiovascular outcomes in diabetic patients with acute myocardial infarction. *J Clin Endocrinol Metab* 95:4993–5002.

Zhou H, Tran PO, Yang S, Zhang T, Le Roy E, Oseid E, Robertson RP. 2004. Regulation of alpha-cell function by the beta-cell during hypoglycemia in Wistar rats: the "switch-off" hypothesis. *Diabetes* 53:1482–1487.

Zhou H, Zhang T, Harmon JS, Bryan J, Robertson RP. 2007. Zinc, not insulin, regulates the rat alpha cell to hypoglycemia in vivo. *Diabetes* 56:1107–1112.

Zoungas S, Patel A, Chalmers J, de Galan BE, Li Q, Billot L., Woodward M, Nimomiya T, Neal B, MacMahon S, Grobbee DE, Kengne AP, Marre M, Heller S and the ADVANCE Collaborative Group. 2010. Severe hypoglycemia and risks of vascular events and death. *N Engl J Med* 363:1410–1418.

Index

Note: Page numbers followed by *f* refer to figures. Page numbers followed by *t* refer to tables. Page numbers in **bold** indicate an in-depth discussion.

A

B

E

W

Y